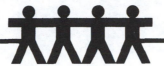

Developing Professional Behaviors

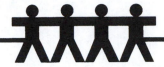

Developing Professional Behaviors

Jack Kasar, PhD, OTR/L
Chair, Department of Occupational Therapy
University of Scranton
Scranton, Pennsylvania

E. Nelson Clark, MS, OTR/L
Private Practice in Mental Health,
Drug and Alcohol Counselor
Hollidaysburg, Pennsylvania

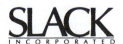

6900 Grove Road • Thorofare, NJ 08086

ISBN: 978-1-55642-316-1

Published by: SLACK Incorporated
              6900 Grove Road
              Thorofare, NJ 08086 USA
              Telephone: 856-848-1000
              Fax: 856-848-6091
              www.slackbooks.com

Contact SLACK Incorporated for more information about other books in this field or about the availability of our books from distributors outside the United States.

Library of Congress Cataloging-in-Publication Data
Developing Professional Behaviors/Jack Kasar, E. Nelson Clark [editors].
        p.cm.
      Includes bibliographical references and index.
      ISBN 1-55642-316-0 (alk. paper)
        1. Physicians--Professional Ethics. 2. Medical personnel--Moral and ethical aspects. 3. Medical ethics. I. Kasar, Jack. II. Clark, E, Nelson.
      R724.D476 2000
      610.69--dc21   99-057166

Printed in the United States of America.

Last digit is print number: 10 9 8 7 6

Dedication

This book is dedicated to those students, practitioners,
and educators with the attitudes, values, and beliefs
that guide them to behave ethically and professionally
in the service of others.

Contents

Dedication v

Acknowledgments xi

About the Editors xiii

Contributing Authors xv

Introduction xvii

PART ONE: Behind the Scenes: Background and Underlying Factors

Chapter One: The Meaning of Professionalism 3

Jack Kasar, PhD, OTR/L

Definition

Professionalism in a Variety of Disciplines

Professionalism in Nursing

Professionalism in Occupational Therapy

Professional Behaviors

Chapter Two: Guiding Ethics 11

Elizabeth Kanny, PhD, OTR/L

Ethics and Values

Major Ethical Principles

Major Ethical Theories

Moral Development

Ethical Problem-Solving

Developing Professionalism

Chapter Three: Developmental Framework 19

Mary E. Muscari, PhD, CRNP, CS

Novice

Apprentice

Expert

Looking into the Future

PART TWO: The Right Stuff: Professional Behaviors

Chapter Four: Dependability 29

Paul Petersen, PhD, OTR/L

Dependability Defined

Significance

Background

How Dependability is Developed

Case Stories/Anecdotal Vignettes

Exercises to Develop Dependability

Chapter Five: Professional Presentation 45

Jan Larkey

Seven Seconds to Image Impact

Body Language

Looking Professional

The Blink Test

Exercises for Professional Presentation

Chapter Six: Initiative 55

Threese A. Clark, MS, OTR/L

Definitions

Background

Extrinsic vs. Intrinsic Initiative/Motivation
Development of Initiative/Motivation
Methods and Ideas

Chapter Seven: Empathy 65
Marian L. Farrell, PhD, RNC
Mary E. Muscari, PhD, CRNP, CS
Background
Developing Empathy
Demonstrating Empathy
Levels of Development
Case Stories/Anecdotal Vignettes
Exercises to Develop Empathy

Chapter Eight: Cooperation..75
Marlene J. Morgan, MOT, OTR/L
Cooperation in Teams and Groups
Development of Cooperative Teams
Roles of Members
Developing Skills
Teamwork and Career Development
Exercises to Develop Cooperation

Chapter Nine: Organization 83
E. Nelson Clark, MS, OTR/L
The Need for Organization
The Function of Organization
Organization as Meaningful Order
Capacity for Delay
The Organized Individual
An Organizational Task

Chapter Ten: Clinical Reasoning...91
Threese A. Clark, MS, OTR/L
Significance
Background
Nature of Clinical Reasoning
Development of Clinical Reasoning
Levels of Development
Methods and Ideas

Chapter Eleven: Supervisory Process 103
Sherry L. Pfister, AAS, COTA/L
Barbara Tennent-Ponterio, MS, OTR/L
Learning Supervision
Behavioral Style Questionnaire
Supervisory Qualities
Management Styles
Novice to Master Supervision
Exercise for Supervisory Process

Chapter Twelve: Verbal Communication 119
Evelyn Anne Mocek, OTR/L, CHT
E. Nelson Clark, MS, OTR/L
Model of Communication
How Do We Communicate?

Types of Communication
Practical Application of Verbal Communication Skills
Health Care Communication
Developing Verbal Communication Awareness

Chapter Thirteen: Written Communication 131
   Mary E. Muscari, PhD, CRNP, CS
   Background
   Developing Written Communication Skills
   Expressive Writing: Client Charting
   Transactional Writing: Formal Papers and Manuscripts
   Levels of Development
   Exercises for Written Communication

PART THREE: **Measuring Up:** *The Professional Development Assessment*

Chapter Fourteen: Development of the Instrument, and its Academic and Clinical Applications 145
   Jack Kasar, PhD, OTR/L
   Assessment of Professional Values and Behaviors
   Development of the Instrument
   Initial Validity and Reliability Information
   Professional Development Assessment©
   Academic and Clinical Applications
   Strategies for Developing Professional Behaviors

PART FOUR: **Full Circle: Developing Professionalism in the Next Generation**

Chapter Fifteen: Learning and Teaching Approaches 157
   Diane E. Watson, MBA, OTR/L, BCP
   Communities, Students, and Professional Education Programs
   Defining Behavioral Expectations and Measuring Performance
   Congruence with Values and Principles Advocated by the Profession
   Congruence with Program Mission, Objectives, and Curriculum Model
   Communicating Performance Expectations
   Instructional Methods

Chapter Sixteen: Continuing Education 165
   Paul Petersen, PhD, OTR/L
   Background
   Continuing Education
   Before You Leave
   During the Course
   After You Return

PART FIVE: **Reality Rehearsal: Structured Activities for Professional Behaviors**©
   Jack Kasar, PhD, OTR/L
   E. Nelson Clark, MS, OTR/L
   Structured Activity #1—Be Careful What You Write© 179
   Structured Activity #2—Judging Books by Their Cover© 183
   Structured Activity #3—Build a Better Mousetrap© 187
   Structured Activity #4—Being on Time© 191
   Structured Activity #5—What do I Say When I Talk to You?© 195
   Structured Activity #6—Seeking the Self© 199
   Structured Activity #7—How Much Do I Really Want It?© 203
   Structured Activity #8—Who Am I and Where Am I Going?© 207

Appendix 211

     Professional Development Assessment©

     Professional Development Assessment Rating Summary Form©

     Professional Behaviors Feedback Form©

Index 217

Laboratory Safety: General Guidelines

1. Notify your instructor immediately if you are pregnant, color blind, allergic to any insect or chemicals, taking immunosuppressive drugs, or have any other medical condition (such as diabetes, immunologic defect) that may require special precautionary measures in the laboratory.

2. Upon entering the laboratory, place all books, coats, purses, backpacks, etc. in designated areas, not on the bench tops.

3. Locate and, when appropriate, learn to use exits, fire extinguisher, fire blanket, chemical shower, eyewash, first aid kit, broken glass container, and cleanup materials for spills.

4. In case of fire, evacuate the room and assemble outside the building.

5. Do not eat, drink, smoke, or apply cosmetics in the laboratory.

6. Confine long hair, loose clothing, and dangling jewelry.

7. Wear shoes at all times in the laboratory.

8. Cover any cuts or scrapes with a sterile, waterproof bandage before attending lab.

9. Wear eye protection when working with chemicals.

10. Never pipet by mouth. Use mechanical pipeting devices.

11. Wash skin immediately and thoroughly if contaminated by chemicals or microorganisms.

12. Do not perform unauthorized experiments.

13. Do not use equipment without instruction.

14. Report all spills and accidents to your instructor immediately.

15. Never leave heat sources unattended.

16. When using hot plates, note that there is no visible sign that they are hot (such as a red glow). Always assume that hot plates are hot.

17. Use an appropriate apparatus when handling hot glassware.

18. Keep chemicals away from direct heat or sunlight.

19. Keep containers of alcohol, acetone, and other flammable liquids away from flames.

20. Do not allow any liquid to come into contact with electrical cords. Handle electrical connectors with dry hands. Do not attempt to disconnect electrical equipment that crackles, snaps, or smokes.

21. Upon completion of laboratory exercises, place all materials in the disposal areas designated by your instructor.

22. Do not pick up broken glassware with your hands. Use a broom and dustpan and discard the glass in designated glass waste containers; never discard with paper waste.

23. Wear disposable gloves when working with blood, other body fluids, or mucous membranes. Change gloves after possible contamination and wash hands immediately after gloves are removed.

24. The disposal symbol indicates that items that may have come in contact with body fluids should be placed in your lab's designated container. It also refers to liquid wastes that should not be poured down the drain into the sewage system.

25. Leave the laboratory clean and organized for the next student.

26. Wash your hands with liquid or powdered soap prior to leaving the laboratory.

27. The biohazard symbol indicates procedures that may pose health concerns.

The caution symbol points out instruments, substances, and procedures that require special attention to safety. These symbols appear throughout this manual.

Measurement Conversions

Metric to American Standard	American Standard to Metric
Length	
1 mm = 0.039 inches	1 inch = 2.54 cm
1 cm = 0.394 inches	1 foot = 0.305 m
1 m = 3.28 feet	1 yard = 0.914 m
1 m = 1.09 yards	1 mile = 1.61 km
Volume	
1 mL = 0.0338 fluid ounces	1 fluid ounce = 29.6 mL
1 L = 4.23 cups	1 cup = 237 mL
1 L = 2.11 pints	1 pint = 0.474 L
1 L = 1.06 quarts	1 quart = 0.947 L
1 L = 0.264 gallons	1 gallon = 3.79 L
Mass	
1 mg = 0.0000353 ounces	1 ounce = 28.3 g
1 g = 0.0353 ounces	1 pound = 0.454 kg
1 kg = 2.21 pounds	

Temperature

To convert temperature:

$$°C = \frac{5}{9}(F - 32) \qquad °F = \frac{9}{5} + 32$$

°F °C

- 230 — 110
- 220
- 210 — 100 ← Water boils
- 200
- 190 — 90
- 180 — 80
- 170
- 160 — 70
- 150
- 140 — 60
- 130
- 120 — 50
- 110
- 100 — 40
- **98.6°F** → ← **37°C**

Normal human body temperature (98.6°F) / Normal human body temperature (37°C)

- 90
- 80 — 30
- 70 — 20
- 60
- 50 — 10
- 40
- 30 — 0 ← Water freezes
- 20
- 10 — −10
- 0
- −10 — −20
- −20 — −30
- −30
- −40 — −40

Centimeters | Inches

- 20 — 8
- 19 — 7
- 18
- 17
- 16 — 6
- 15
- 14
- 13 — 5
- 12
- 11 — 4
- 10
- 9 — 3
- 8
- 7
- 6 — 2
- 5
- 4 — 1
- 3
- 2
- 1
- 0 — 0

Acknowledgments

We would like to express thanks to the students, staff, and faculty who helped us to focus on the assessment and development of professional behaviors. I would like to particularly mention Marjorie Scaffa at the University of South Alabama for pilot testing the instrument and contributing data, together with Mount Aloysius College and the University of Scranton.

A special note of consideration is given to the contributors who worked and struggled through the process of bringing professional behaviors down to earth and conveying them in practical terms.

A number of student research assistants at the University of Scranton deserve recognition, including Mary Beckish, Rachel Budney, and Alison Devers for data entry and analysis, and library research; and Jill Beckish and Shannon Kelder for assisting with proofreading this manuscript.

Appreciation is extended to John Bond and Amy Drummond for believing in the idea and the need for such a work, and to Lauren Plummer for layout design and copy-editing. Finally, gratitude is given to Debra Christy, at SLACK Incorporated, for supporting and following this project through to successful completion.

About the Editors

Jack Kasar, PhD, OTR/L

Jack Kasar is the founding chairman of the Department of Occupational Therapy at the University of Scranton. He received a B.A. in Psychology from West Chester University, a Master of Science in Occupational Therapy from the Medical College of Virginia-Virginia Commonwealth University, and a Doctorate of Philosophy from the University of Pennsylvania.

Dr. Kasar has been involved in the field of Occupational Therapy for over 25 years. He was an officer in the U.S. Navy Medical Service Corps, and has held several clinical positions, including Director of Occupational Therapy Services at White Haven Center.

For the past 15 years, Dr. Kasar has worked in the area of Occupational Therapy education and has held the positions of Program Director and Clinical Education Coordinator. He has taught course work in Human Development, Occupational Therapy Theory, Kinesiology, Neuroanatomy, and Occupational Therapy Practice courses in Developmental Disabilities and in Physical Rehabilitation.

Dr. Kasar is a member of the American Occupational Therapy Association, World Federation of Occupational Therapists, the Pennsylvania Occupational Therapy Association, and Sensory Integration International. His research interests include: curriculum development, sensory integration and neurological approaches, functional assessments, and in particular, the development of professional behaviors.

E. Nelson Clark, MS, OTR/L

Nelson Clark began his professional career in the U.S. Air Force during the Vietnam Conflict as an administrative, personnel, and recruiter technician. He completed a Bachelor of Science degree in Occupational Therapy at the University of Missouri, and following graduation accepted a commission as an officer in the U.S. Navy Medical Service Corps.

Nelson served as a staff occupational therapist and department head in many areas, including psychiatry, hand therapy, orthotics, and special needs children. He received a Master of Science in Occupational Therapy from the University of San Jose. He eventually attained the position of Specialty Section Advisor for Occupational Therapy to the Naval Surgeon General.

Following retirement from the military, Nelson entered academics and was Program Director of the Associate Degree program for Occupational Therapy Assistants at Mount Aloysius College for 7 years. During this time, he served for 4 years as a Division Director for Allied Health.

Nelson has authored and edited a number of books, journal articles, and manuals. As an inventor, he has been awarded two patents for products that are being marketed successfully. He received the Maddock Award twice for his contributions to the profession of Occupational Therapy. Nelson is currently in private practice as a counselor, and is planning to operate and manage his own business, a small golf course, which is scheduled to open in the Spring of 2000.

Contributing Authors

Threese A. Clark, MS, OTR/L
Chair
Occupational Therapy Program
Mount Aloysius College
Cresson, Pennsylvania

Marian L. Farrell, PhD, RNC
Associate Professor
Department of Nursing
University of Scranton
Scranton, Pennsylvania

Jan Larkey
Author of Flatter Your Figure
Speaker, Consultant
Pittsburgh, Pennsylvania

Elizabeth Kanny, PhD, OTR/L
Chair
Division of Occupational Therapy
Department of Rehabilitation Medicine
University of Washington
Seattle, Washington

Evelyn Anne Mocek, OTR/L, CHT
Instructor
Occupational Therapy Assistant Program
Mount Aloysius College
Cresson, Pennsylvania

Marlene J. Morgan, MOT, OTR/L
Instructor
Department of Occupational Therapy
University of Scranton
Scranton, Pennsylvania

Mary E. Muscari, PhD, CRNP, CS
Associate Professor
Department of Nursing
University of Scranton
Scranton, Pennsylvania

Paul Petersen, PhD, OTR/L
Contract Therapist
St. Joseph Hospital
Lancaster, Pennsylvania

Sherry L. Pfister, AAS, COTA/L
Clinical Education Coordinator
Occupational Therapy Assistant Program
Mount Aloysius College
Cresson, Pennsylvania

Barbara Tennent-Ponterio, MS, OTR/L
Director of Occupational Therapy
IHS at Mountain View Nursing Center
Greensburg, Pennsylvania

Diane E. Watson, MBA, OTR/L, BCP
Doctoral Candidate
University of Toronto
Clinical Education Coordinator (formerly)
Department of Occupational Therapy
University of Scranton
Scranton, Pennsylvania

Introduction

The Need for Professionalism

In recent years there has been an increasing need to actively focus attention on the development of professional behaviors in students and practitioners of health care professions at all levels. Behaviors such as professional demeanor, teamwork, organizational skills, empathy, initiative, and dependability are highly valued. Students and beginning practitioners are expected to be responsible, appropriately assertive, and self-motivated, as well as able to function relatively independently with some guidance. These behaviors cannot be taken for granted. The development of professional skills in students and clinicians requires practice, experience, role mentorship, and evaluative feedback.

The teaching of professional behaviors has mainly been accomplished through the role modeling approach. Inherent in this perspective is the implicit assumption that acting professionally is automatically assimilated. Today, one cannot assume that these qualities are innately present. Therefore, they cannot be taken for granted. Professional behaviors must be developed and nurtured not only because we value them and think that they're important to have, but because they embody what it takes to be successful as a professional. It is part of our responsibility of fostering professional socialization as students, practitioners, and educators. It is also necessary to survive in an ever-changing, evolving, and dynamic market place. Additionally, it is what is ultimately required to create and ensure a vibrant practice environment focused on the clients and consumers that are served.

This work on the broad topic of professionalism and professional behaviors is directed primarily toward students, but should also prove useful to clinicians and educators in the health care professions. This project and now this book were undertaken in the hopes that it would stimulate thinking and reflection on professional aspects, and that it would provide an approach to assist in assessing and developing professional behaviors in students and clinicians. Developing professionalism and professional behaviors needs to be a conscious, active and deliberate process on the part of students, practitioners, and educators.

The book is divided into five sections. The first two sections deal with professionalism generally, and how to develop specific behaviors. In Part I, Chapter 1, background information is provided on the meaning and definition of professional behaviors as related to a number of professions; in Chapter 2, the guiding ethics that underlie professionalism and drive the professional behaviors are discussed; and in Chapter 3 a theoretical framework is proposed as a model to use in helping to grow professionalism.

Part II begins the main body of the book, and is divided into individual chapters that focus on an expanded treatment of the general categories of professional behaviors. The organization of this section of the book is based on the 10 behavioral categories included in the *Professional Development Assessment* (see Chapter 14 and Appendix). The assessment encompasses many of the behaviors discussed under the broader topic of professionalism. These behaviors are woven through earlier and later sections of the book, and provide an underlying framework and consistent point of reference. The behavioral categories include: dependability, professional presentation, initiative, empathy, cooperation, organization, clinical reasoning, supervisory process, verbal communication, and written communication. Each chapter covers in varying degrees a definition of the behavior and its significance, background information, how it develops, and approaches or mini-exercises to enhance the behavior. The assessment and the behavioral categories are by no means an all-inclusive list of the aspects of professionalism, but are intended to represent and reflect the areas of importance and concern most often cited by students, practitioners, and educators.

The third and fourth sections provide information and relate to the health care professions students as they move on in their careers to become accomplished practitioners, supervisors, and educators. Part III reviews the development of the *Professional Development Assessment,* initial validity and reliability information, and how the instrument has been used in academic and clinical settings. Part IV explores how to develop professionalism in oneself and others as part of the next generation, and includes chapters on learning and teaching approaches, as well as continuing education.

In Part V there is a collection of structured activities for professional behaviors devised for self-use and/or with small groups. The appendix includes a copy of the *Professional Development Assessment* and related materials.

It is hoped that this work will offer relevant information, provide useful tools to assess and develop professional behaviors, and stimulate further investigation into this important area of concern for health care professionals.

Jack Kasar, PhD, OTR/L
E. Nelson Clark, MS, OTR/L

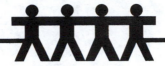

Part One

Behind the Scenes: Background and Underlying Factors

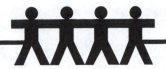

Chapter One

The Meaning of Professionalism

Jack Kasar, PhD, OTR/L

This chapter will provide general background information on the meaning and definition of professional behaviors as related to a number of professions. As mentioned in the introduction, a large part of the broader organization of the book is based on the behavioral categories found in the *Professional Development Assessment* (see Chapter 14 and Appendix). The assessment includes many of the behaviors considered under the general topic of professionalism. These behaviors and related aspects are integrated through each section of the book and serve to provide an underlying, consistent point of reference and framework. The behavioral categories, in the order they appear on the assessment, include: dependability, professional presentation, initiative, empathy, cooperation, organization, clinical reasoning, supervisory process, verbal communication, and written communication (Kasar, Clark, Watson, & Pfister, 1996). The assessment and behavioral categories are not intended as an all-inclusive list of aspects of professionalism, but rather they represent areas of importance and concern most often cited by students, practitioners, and educators.

Before discussing the definition and meaning of professionalism, a review of the current trends that accentuate the importance of professional behaviors is in order. With the shift from old to new paradigms within the current practice environment, there is an increasing need for high caliber technical skills and professional behaviors. Previously the practice orientation was focused on models that were institutionally based and illness-oriented. The practitioner was guided toward independence and maintenance of quality assurance.

Consumer awareness, rapid advances in technology and far-reaching changes in the monetary reimbursement system have created the need for change. Currently, the practice of health-related professions is more consumer and community focused, with an emphasis on wellness and prevention. The practitioner is now encouraged to be more interdependent and concerned with quality enhancement, rather than just the status quo. These changes are intended to promote practitioner accountability, while providing the most efficient, cost effective approach to consumer focused treatment. Table 1-1 summarizes some of the changes in the practice environment.

The changes in the practice environment have influenced professional preparation in a number of ways. In the past, teaching methods created a passive learning environment. The emphasis in both academic and clinical settings was on content issues and rote memorization. Today, there is a need to develop active, responsible, life-long learners, whether they are students or clinicians. While content issues are still significant, the exponential growth in new knowledge changes the focus to greater concentration on thinking and interacting. Therefore, great importance and concern has to be placed on clinical reasoning and professional behaviors for all practitioners. Table 1-2 summarizes some of the changes in professional preparation.

With the changes in the practice environment and professional preparation emphasizing the importance of pro-

Table 1-1

PRACTICE ENVIRONMENT

OLD PARADIGM	NEW PARADIGM
Institutional/Medical Model	Community Based/Consumer Focused
Disease/Disability Perspective	Wellness/Prevention
Individual/Facility Providers	Team/Regional Group Providers
Quality Assurance	Quality Improvement
Independent Professional Practice	Interdependent Directed and Managed Services

Table 1-2

PROFESSIONAL PREPARATION

OLD PARADIGM	NEW PARADIGM
Lecture and Listen	Inquiry and Active Participation
Textbook	Interactive Multimedia
Rote Memorization	Problem-Based Approach
Emphasis on Content	Focus on Process
Teacher Directed	Teacher Facilitated and Learner Self-Directed

fessionalism and professional behaviors, take a look at the traditional definition of a profession.

Definition

According to Miller and Keane (1987), "A profession continuously enlarges its body of knowledge, functions autonomously in formulation of policy, and maintains by force of organization or concerted opinion high standards of achievement and conduct. Members of a profession are committed to continuing study, place service above personal gain, and are committed to providing practical services vital to human and social welfare" (p. 1014).

Another publication focuses on the prestigious aspects of the term *profession* as follows: "one of a limited number of occupations or vocations involving special learning and carrying a certain social prestige, especially the learned professions: law, medicine and the Church" (Lexicon Publications, 1989, p. 798).

O'Rourke (1989) broadly defined a profession by suggesting that there are three dimensions that all groups must follow. The first is a normative dimension that includes values and ethics supporting the idea of self-regulation. The second is an evaluative dimension that includes overseeing standards of practice and guiding professional activity. Finally, there is a cognitive dimension that includes standards for education and demonstration of mastery of appropriate practice skills and clinical applications. Creek and Ormston (1996) speak about occupational therapy (OT) consisting of three essential elements: philosophy, practice, and theory that must be linked closely together. These elements apply to almost any profession, and professional practice in particular is "the purposeful application of knowledge, skills and techniques to achieve predefined goals, utilizing compatible frameworks and models that do not compromise the shared value system" (p. 7).

The formal definitions speak to advanced learning, personal responsibility, enhanced prestige, high standards of performance and behavior, and self-regulation. How does this reflect itself in professionalism and professional behaviors? I would like to examine briefly how a number of professions have viewed acting professionally.

Professionalism in a Variety of Disciplines

A number of related disciplines have identified the need for and the importance of professionalism and developing professional behaviors. Educators in many professions (such as scientists, health specialists, nurses, physicians, and teachers) have emphasized the value and need of proactively enhancing professional skills.

Schwen (1988) discussed virtuous behavior and described it as characteristic behavior that reflects the commonly held values and beliefs of a profession and could be promulgated by professional organizations. Further, it was strongly suggested that desired behaviors need to be well-understood, explicitly stated, and modeled to benefit the profession. Verhulst, Colliver, Paiva, and Williams (1984) developed a questionnaire and surveyed supervisors of graduate physicians in the residency phase of their education. Principal component data analysis yielded two distinct factors that represented a clinical skills dimension and a professional behavior dimension. The findings suggested that when considering desirability and being chosen as a personal physician, the supervisors viewed clinical skills and professional behavior as being of equal importance. However, when they looked at overall competence and correlated it with the two factors, clinical skills were seen as slightly more important than professional behaviors. This suggests that resident supervisors were a little more concerned with clinical competence as opposed to how the residents behaved professionally. Reynolds (1994), on the other hand, proposed that the development of professionalism in physicians needed to be purposeful and proactive. He suggested further that mentoring and role modeling be used together with a curriculum-long program to develop and evaluate professionalism and professional conduct.

Gauld (1982) considered science education and the development of a scientific attitude and noted that the aspects that embodied the scientific attitude were desirable for all to possess. Some of these aspects, such as open-mindedness, objectivity, accuracy, and intellectual honesty, are analogous to professional behaviors. It was proposed that those who held the scientific attitude would be more considerate of others and their point of view, and would be able to live and work more cooperatively with other individuals. Spruill and Benshoff (1996) discuss the development of professionalism in graduate counseling students and suggest that professionalism is a continuous process that pertains to all professionals. It needs to begin in graduate programs and requires the opportunity for modeling, practice, and sponsorship from professionals and professional organizations.

Professionalism in Nursing

The nursing profession, more than any other discipline, has concerned itself with the issue of professional values and behaviors. A recent study compared ratings of the importance of professional nursing values of faculty with that of students, and found that faculty rated the importance of behaviors significantly higher than did students (Eddy, Elfrink, Weis, & Schank, 1994). In particular, the faculty valued equality, human dignity, and freedom greater than did the students.

In an earlier study, again comparing faculty and student ratings of values, faculty ratings of professional values were higher than student ratings (Thurston, Flood, Shupe, & Gerald, 1989). However, in the same study ratings of personal values were similar between faculty and students, supporting the contention that individuals are attracted to a profession by what they believe it represents and how they perceive that their skills and abilities are suited to that field.

Weis, Schank, Eddy, and Elfrink (1993) compared program objectives for a number of nursing curricula to determine how well they included the essential values and behaviors espoused by the American Association of Colleges of Nursing (AACN). The essential values included: altruism, equality, aesthetics, freedom, human dignity, justice, and truth. They found that most of the professional behaviors were evident in program objectives. However, the values of truth and aesthetics were only minimally represented in stated outcomes for the program. It was further noted that while values were often learned in an informal fashion, it was proposed that they be included as part of the formal content. Elfrink and Lutz (1991) surveyed 697 undergraduate nurse educators concerning the seven essential professional values identified by the AACN. The findings suggested that the large majority of respondents viewed the values as aspects that nurses need in practice, and as such should be part of the curriculum.

Miller, Adams, and Beck (1993) developed a self-rating behavioral inventory to assess professional behaviors in nurses. Their inventory took a different slant than the AACN measure and included more general, broader aspects in their view of professionalism, such as educational background, communication and publication, community service, and research involvement.

Professionalism in Occupational Therapy

Periodically, individuals within the field of occupational therapy have focused on the development of professional behaviors. Opacich and Hughes (1990) examined professional behaviors in OT graduates during the first year of employment. A scale was used that looked at 17 attributes and rated students from poor to superior. Some of the behaviors assessed included judgement, leadership, technical repertoire, and professional identity. Crist (1986) cited that a key method to develop professional roles during fieldwork was through modeling, especially since new behaviors are taught and existing behaviors modified in this manner. Sabari (1985) focused on the importance of the process of professional socialization to OT educators and emphasized the need to actively facilitate professional socialization. A nursing study also supports these ideas, with the contention that developing professional values needs to be an important part of professional socialization (Schank and Weis, 1989). They suggest that clinical experience is more essential to value development than the classroom, and that professional identity is really solidified in the clinic.

In the *Guide to Fieldwork Education* (AOTA, 1991), a document from the Department of Rehabilitation Medicine at the Michael Reese Hospital cited that the development of essential professional behaviors in the student therapist is an important part of the fieldwork experience. Sands (1995) developed an approach for required student conferences as a means of providing formative feedback to students on personal attitudes and behaviors. Some of the categories discussed were attitude, interpersonal skills, time management, and problem-solving abilities. The intent was to increase student self-awareness through self-assessment, and thereby positively influence areas needing growth.

The final performance subcategory of the Fieldwork Evaluation (AOTA, 1991), Administration/Professionalism, assessed in a general way several aspects of professionalism, including: managing time effectively, participating in the supervisory relationship, and assuming responsibility for professional behavior and growth. Kautzmann (1984) developed a Likert-type scale to provide feedback on professional behavior during Level I fieldwork. The behaviors assessed were more specific and definitive, e.g., asking for help or information appropri-

ately, and participating in clinical problem-solving with the therapist. It was found that students valued and used the feedback.

Breines (1988), in an attempt to redefine professionalism for OT, suggested that one needs to possess a caring attitude, a desire for life-long learning, a dedication to teaching others, and a concern for both giving and receiving pertinent educational information. Fidler (1996) noted that professional development involves learning and personal growth that goes beyond the mastery of related knowledge and technology that are part of a discipline. It is essential that a professional acquires a regard for the dynamics of human relationships and interpersonal skills. In order to develop these abilities one needs to integrate attitudes, beliefs, and values that reflect personal integrity, demonstrate an empathetic regard for others, show a respect for different points of view, and possess a sense of responsibility to contribute to the welfare of others (Fidler, 1996). Jenkins and Brotherton (1995) suggested that the idea of democratic professionalism is based on the client/practitioner relationship, and that there needs to be a decentralization of expert knowledge and mutual valuing of the experience and knowledge of the participants.

Professional Behaviors

Professional behaviors and their development are timely and important topics. As noted at the beginning, in this particular work the behaviors on which we focus are dependability, professional presentation, initiative, empathy, cooperation, organization, clinical reasoning, supervisory process, verbal communication, and written communication (Kasar, et al., 1996). A few initial comments on each of the behaviors will now be cited.

Dependability — Health care professionals are expected to be on time and responsible in carrying out their duties and responding to client/patient needs. Functioning as a member of a health care team requires participants to meet deadlines and adhere to schedules.

Professional Presentation — Demeanor, professional presentation, and manner are essential and highly valued. Students, like practitioners, are expected to present themselves in a way that is accepted by peers, clients, and employers. Genuine interest in providing your services to others is demonstrated through focused attention and positive regard.

Initiative — Employers are increasingly requiring their employees to be highly motivated and self-directed.

Valued employees are the ones who demonstrate a positive, energetic, and motivated manner. They take responsibility for starting projects and contribute to the development and enhancement of programs and services.

Empathy — An important and necessary prerequisite to building therapeutic relationships is empathy. In order to establish empathic relationships, you must demonstrate the ability to listen, understand, share, and be sensitive to another person's perceptions of a situation.

Cooperation — In the health care industry today, teamwork is a way of life. Health care professionals will need to work collaboratively in interdisciplinary, multidisciplinary, and transdisciplinary teams. The health care environment requires individuals to be cooperative, flexible, and adaptable.

Organization — The quality and efficiency of your services as a professional are improved by your organizational abilities. Clients/patients and colleagues will often make value assessments of the service you are providing based on the perception of how well you are organized. Also, how well a team performs is inherently dependent upon the organizational abilities of its members.

Clinical Reasoning — The dynamic process of inquiry that takes place within the context of clinical practice is called clinical reasoning. Problem-solving skills, knowledge, and experience are needed to reason through problems encountered in practice situations. Students are required to enhance and refine their problem-solving and critical-thinking skills in order to develop clinical reasoning abilities.

Supervisory Process — Health care professionals need to make use of the supervisory process, and must be ready to give and receive constructive and productive feedback. They are expected to serve as mentors for newcomers to their profession, as well as to work positively with assistants, aides, and other professionals. Interpersonal and supervisory abilities are required to guide and mentor others.

Verbal Communication — Verbal proficiency is one of the most outward personal traits of a professional that can be used to market your service and your profession. Being articulate will certainly have a positive influence on your clients/patients, colleagues, and employer. Health care professionals are required, and students are expected, to make contributions to discussions at staffings, conferences, rounds, inservices, and other pertinent meetings.

Written Communication — Writing is the most important non-verbal personal trait of a professional that can be used to market your service and your profession. In the health care industry today, written documents must be produced according to a particular institution's standards and must stand up to review and scrutiny by departments, facilities, quality assurers, third party payers, and the legal system.

Professional behaviors cannot be taken for granted and it cannot be assumed that they are innately present. Professional behaviors must be nurtured and developed in students and clinicians because they embody what it takes to be successful as a professional and what it takes to survive in an ever-changing, evolving, and dynamic practice environment. The balance of this section will focus on the underlying and guiding ethics upon which professional behaviors are based, and a theoretical framework that can be used to help enhance the growth of professionalism and professional behaviors in health care practitioners.

References

American Occupational Therapy Association. (1991). *Guide to fieldwork education.* Rockville, MD: Author.

Breines, E. B. (1988). Redefining professionalism for occupational therapy. *American Journal of Occupational Therapy, 42(1),* 55-57.

Creek, J., & Ormston, C. (1996). The essential elements of professional motivation. *British Journal of Occupational Therapy, 59(1),* 7-10.

Crist, P. H. (1986). *Contemporary issues in clinical education.* Thorofare, NJ: SLACK Incorporated.

Eddy, D. M., Elfrink, V., Weis, D., & Schank, M. J. (1994). Importance of professional nursing values: A national study of baccalaureate programs. *Journal of Nursing Education, 33,* 257-262.

Elfrink, V., & Lutz, E. M. (1991). American association of colleges of nursing essential values: National study of faculty perceptions, practices, and plans. *Journal of Professional Nursing, 7,* 239-245.

Fidler, G. (1996). Developing a repertoire of professional behaviors. *American Journal of Occupational Therapy, 50(7),* 583-587.

Gauld, C. (1982). The scientific attitude and science education: A critical review. *Science Education, 66,* 109-121.

Jenkins, M., & Brotherton, C. (1995). Implications of a theoretical framework for practice. *British Journal of Occupational Therapy, 58(9),* 392-396.

Kasar, J., Clark, N., Watson, D., & Pfister, S. (1996). *Professional Development Assessment.* Unpublished form.

Kautzmann, L. (1984). *The development of guidelines for feedback on professional behavior in level I field work performance.* Unpublished doctoral dissertation, Nova University, Milwaukee, WI.

Lexicon Publications (1989). *The new lexicon webster's dictionary of the english language.* New York, NY: Lexicon Publications, Inc.

Miller, B. F., & Keane, C. B. (1987). *Encyclopedia and dictionary of medicine, nursing, and allied health.* Philadelphia, PA: W. B. Saunders.

Miller, B. K., Adams, D., & Beck, L. (1993). A behavioral inventory for professionalism in nursing. *Journal of Professional Nursing, 9,* 290-295.

O'Rourke, M. W. (1989). Generic professional behaviors: Implications for the clinical nurse specialist role. *Clinical Nurse Specialist, 3(3),* 128-132.

Opacich, K. J., & Hughes, C. J. (1990). *Employer assessment of performance and professional development.* Paper presented at Commission on Education, American Occupational Therapy Association annual meeting, New Orleans, LA.

Reynolds, P. P. (1994). Reaffirming professionalism through the education community. *Annals of Internal Medicine, 120(7),* 609-614.

Sabari, J. S. (1985). Professional socialization: Implications for occupational therapy education. *American Journal of Occupational Therapy, 39,* 96-102.

Sands, M. (1995). Readying occupational therapy assistant students for level II fieldwork: Beyond academics to personal behaviors and attitudes. *American Journal of Occupational Therapy, 49,* 150-152.

Schwen, T. M. (1988). *Professional ethics: An analysis of some arguments for development of virtuous behavior.* Paper presented at the annual meeting of the Association for Educational Communications and Technology, New Orleans, LA.

Schank, M. J., & Weis, D. (1989). A study of values of baccalaureate nursing students and graduate nurses from a secular and a nonsecular program. *Journal of Professional Nursing, 5(1),* 17-22.

Spruill, D. A., & Benshoff, J. M. (1996). The future is now: Promoting professionalism among counselors-in-training. *Journal of Counseling and Development, 74,* 468-471.

Thurston, H. I., Flood, M. A., Shupe, I. S., & Gerald, K. B. (1989). Values held by nursing faculty and students in a university setting. *Journal of Professional Nursing, 5,* 199-207.

Verhulst, S. J., Colliver, J. A., Paiva, R. E., & Williams, R. G. (1984). *Dimensions of physician performance during residency.* Paper presented at a meeting of the Evaluation Network/Evaluation Research Society, San Francisco, CA.

Weis, D., Schank, M. J., Eddy, D., & Elfrink, V. (1993). Professional values in baccalaureate nursing education. *Journal of Professional Nursing, 9,* 336-342.

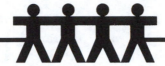

Chapter Two

Guiding Ethics

Elizabeth Kanny, PhD, OTR/L

Ethics underlie just about everything that you will do as a professional. Professional behaviors evolve from your own ethical standards of right and wrong. How we behave and choose to treat others is strongly influenced by our sense of morality. Morality, or ethics, is rooted in the conflicting drives of people to act either selfishly or altruistically (Sieghart, 1985). Moral judgments are based on ideas of how social cooperation should be organized (Rest, 1994). That is, we behave in such a way as to protect the basic human values of our clients and professional colleagues and do the "right" thing. Thus, ethics is actually concerned with right and wrong and how we make decisions regarding how to act.

Ethics and Professionalism

Ethics in professions stem from the Hippocratic Oath (5th Century B.C.), which states that physicians should strive 'for the benefit of the sick and for service to humanity'. Undoubtedly, one of the driving factors that led you to choose a career in health care was your desire to "do good" and help others (altruism). In today's complex and fast-changing health care environment, we are seeing issues that challenge our basic morals, including universal access, reasonable equality of benefits, fairness of burdens, and the quality and efficiency of care (Brody, 1994). As a health care practitioner, you will need to be able to recognize ethical dilemmas, apply problem-solving techniques, and come to a decision, and then act in a way that you believe to be ethical and professional.

Ethical Dilemmas

While you are a student and when you begin practicing in your profession, you will undoubtedly encounter problems that are not solely treatment issues and are not legal issues, but rather fall into another category - ethical dilemmas. Here are some examples:

• You are having lunch with a few classmates and the topic of tests comes up. After some hesitation, one person says that she has observed another classmate looking at other students' papers during tests. Two others chime in saying they have seen the same thing, but have been afraid to mention it. You don't want to "rat" on a fellow student, but think this could be serious. What options do you have?

• One of your classmates has been working the night shift in order to pay for tuition and rent. She comes to you a few days before a paper is due and asks if she could use your paper as an example because she has not had time to start her paper yet and would appreciate a "jump start". What should you say?

• You are doing a clinical internship and are working with a patient who is hospitalized for acute depression related to loss of a job. In the process of therapy, you become attracted to each other and some flirting takes place. He asks you to go out on a date after he is discharged next week. What should you tell him?

• You have just finished your degree and have taken a position with a fast-paced rehabilitation center. On your first day on the job, your supervisor asks you to administer the Peabody Developmental Motor Scales to a child with severe motor impairments. You are familiar with the test, however, you have never administered it to a child. You think to yourself that everyone has to start somewhere and you don't want to disappoint your boss. Should you go ahead and administer the evaluation?

• You go to see a new patient at his bedside, introduce yourself and provide information about why you're seeing him and what services you offer. The patient flatly refuses your services, yet you know that he needs therapy. What do you do?

• An inpatient who has cancer in remission is admitted for a worsening of symptoms. You are seeing her for strengthening, range of motion (ROM) and activities of daily living (ADLs). After a diagnostic work-up by her physician, it is found that her cancer has metastasized and she is not expected to survive for more than 2 months. Do you continue to treat her?

• Included in your overbooked school system caseload is a sixth grader whom you have been seeing for several years. She is emotionally needy and depressed. Although she has reached her original goals, you hesitate to discontinue treatment because she enjoys the individual attention she gets in therapy. You just received four new referrals. Do you stop seeing this student so you can take the new referrals?

• Medicare will not pay a bill because it does not reimburse for maintenance activities. Your supervisor asks you to change your written documentation so that it is reimbursable because the client needs further treatment. What should you do?

• You have been providing home care twice a week for a patient who was discharged from the hospital after having a stroke. He has made progress and now only needs your services once a week. Your supervisor tells you not to reduce your home visits because they are covered by the client's insurance and she wants you to get the maximum reimbursement. What should you do?

These are examples of problems you may face that present ethical dilemmas. When you read these examples, you may feel conflicted, anxious, or feel that something is not right - this may be your sense of 'ethical tension' (Opacich, 1996). Although we spend a lot of time and effort learning and refining our technical skills, we tend to spend less time addressing the ethics and values that shape us as professionals.

The purpose of this chapter is to provide you with information about ethics and ethical dilemmas so you will be better prepared to face situations and decisions that have ethical components. Ethical terms and concepts will be defined and discussed as they relate to professionalism, methods for ethical problem-solving will be presented, and hopefully a sense of responsibility to act in an ethical and professional manner will be supported.

Ethics and Values

Of all the aspects of professionalism, ethics will be one of the most complex in your future role as a health care practitioner. Ethics is the branch of philosophy that concerns itself with morality; right vs. wrong, justice, equality, free will, and responsibility. Ethics are the ways through which we determine right from wrong so that our relationships with people can be harmonious and respectful (Rest, 1994). The goal of morals is to protect those values or goods that we cherish, such as quality of life, property, liberty, or our ideas.

Ethical dilemmas are most usually characterized by the lack of an obvious, agreed-upon, right course of action (Hansen, 1998). This is often called *ethical tension* and can be described as feeling conflicted, having an intuitive discomfort with a situation, or sensing a threat to personal integrity (Opacich, 1996). In these situations, the health care professional must sort out what the real issue is and consider it in light of ethical principles.

Values

It is important for each health professional to know his or her own values, to clarify how they relate to personal and professional life, and to recognize and respect other people's values systems (Purtillo & Haddad, 1996). We each have our own personal ethics that are shaped by religious beliefs, cultural heritage, family values, moral teaching, education, and life experiences (Tourigny, 1992). Societal ethics are a compilation of personal ethics held by various individuals within a society and are reflected in our laws and other societal practices. Professional ethics are influenced and evolved from both personal and societal ethics, but are learned and developed through our professional education and practice (Hansen, 1998; Purtillo, 1993; Tourigny, 1992). Thus, professional ethics represent the values and commitments of our field and provide standards that guide our professional behaviors.

Most professions have identified a set of core values and attitudes that represent their beliefs and general philosophy. Such documents of core values and attitudes usually emanate from historical creeds or pledges (for example, the Nightingale Pledge of 1893 from the nursing profession). Central to most core values documents is respect for people or human dignity (Craven & Hirnle, 1996).

The seven core values for nurses (AACN, 1985) are altruism, equality, esthetics, freedom, human dignity, justice, and truth; those of other health professions are similar.

Professional Codes of Ethics

Ethical codes are common to most professions and address what is called applied normative ethics - the day-to-day deliberations that health care practitioners face about "the right thing to do" (Beauchamp & Childress, 1994). Professional guidelines or codes proscribe or prescribe appropriate ethical and professional behavior based on ethical principles and current legal standards. Generally, professionals are expected to uphold a higher degree of ethical behavior than the general public. In turn, the public grants rights or privileges to the profession beyond those normally granted to all citizens. Professional ethics codes are written in a way that clients', patients', and colleagues' best interests are ensured, and that the public is protected. Compliance with ethical codes is encouraged and enforced. In ethics, the concern is with actual behaviors and their outcomes, rather than with intent. Substandard practices, even if well-intentioned, may damage others.

The general purposes or functions of a professional code of ethics are: to define or articulate the ethical stances and behaviors of the profession, to communicate what is expected of members of the profession, to provide guidance for making ethical decisions, to enhance the recognition and identity of the profession through a sense of common commitment, and to ensure ethical practices to the public (Mosey, 1992; Tourigny, 1992). Health care practitioners should become familiar with their association's code of ethics and enforcement procedures. In addition, if your profession is licensed or certified in your state, there will be ethical regulations that are promulgated and enforced by state law.

Major Ethical Principles

Beauchamp & Childress (1994) identify major ethical principles in health care as autonomy, beneficence, nonmaleficence, and justice. Several other ethical principles related to relationships between practitioners and clients include veracity, fidelity, privacy, and confidentiality (Purtillo, 1993). It is important to understand these principles so that when you engage in analyzing and problem-solving ethical dilemmas you will have a foundation and terminology with which to discuss cases or situations. Understanding the basic ethical principles provides you with a way to articulate your argument or position to others and will give you confidence in taking an ethical stance.

Autonomy

Autonomy is the right of an individual to be self-determining and make independent decisions about one's life (Hansen, 1998). It is the principle of self-governance and pertains to liberty rights, privacy, individual choice, the right to self-determination, and respect for the wishes of a competent person or his or her representative. Health care issues related to autonomy include competency, informed consent, disclosure of information, and acceptance or refusal of medically indicated treatment (Opacich, 1996). Autonomy gives a client or patient the right to make health care decisions based on his or her individual goals and values.

Beneficence

This principle is basic to health care and refers to actions that benefit others and do good (Veatch & Flack, 1997). It implies both actively doing good and considering the potential harm of actions. This means that as professionals we must not only promote good, but also avoid doing harm, prevent harm, and remove harm when it is being inflicted (Beauchamp & Childress, 1994). Doing good for others also involves bringing out what is best for another person.

Nonmaleficence

This principle is fundamental. It means one should not cause harm. The health care practitioner must not inflict harm, but prevent harm and remove harm (Beauchamp

& Childress, 1994). It is important to determine the risks and benefits of an action and to avoid actions that directly cause harm. Issues related to this principle include euthanasia, withdrawing treatment, and quality of life.

Justice

This principle relates to issues of fairness and equitable distribution of goods and services. When choices need to be made, benefits and harms are distributed fairly (Veatch & Flack, 1997). The principle of justice helps us to assign priorities in providing our services, determining fees and payments, and meeting public aid and private insurance criteria. Distributive justice refers to fairness in allocating health care resources. Procedural justice has to do with the process used for ordering things in a fair way. Compensatory justice is the provision of resources to a wronged or injured individual.

Moral Principles Related to Relationships

The principles of veracity, fidelity, confidentiality, and privacy are critical to creating trust and form the basis for the contract between the patient/client and health care practitioner (Opacich, 1996). These principles support autonomy.

Veracity refers to the obligation to tell the truth and not deceive others, honesty with a client or his or her representative, and honesty in reporting the status of clients/patients and services rendered.

Fidelity means being faithful by keeping promises and contracts. This also entails meeting the patient's reasonable expectations (Purtillo, 1993). This means that the client may expect basic respect, competence in your practice, honesty relative to the policies of your place of employment, adherence to patient protection laws, and honor of agreements between yourself and the client (Purtillo, 1993).

Confidentiality pertains to access to personal or private information. Privacy implies limited access to a person and a respect for his or her right to privacy. It means that there are aspects of a person's existence and life into which no one else should intrude. Confidentiality simply means keeping client information within appropriate limits and abiding by rules of consent. It is the longest-standing ethical dictum in health care codes of ethics. The most commonly accepted definition of confidential information is

information about a client that may be harmful, shameful, or embarrassing to that individual (Purtillo, 1993). That information can be verbal (directly from you), written, or electronic data. The client or patient is the best judge of whether the information is sensitive and should be treated confidentially.

Law vs. Ethics

Often we deal with ethical problems through the law. The law is based on the principle of justice. Laws are the formal rules of conduct that govern society. Laws are constantly changing based on court decisions, state and federal statutes, and regulations. In a legal dilemma, arguments for and against a particular case are discussed relative to social values, political forces, and legal precedents. Thus, interpretations of laws may lead to different conclusions in seemingly similar situations, depending on the circumstances of the case and the view of the judge. In today's society, there are a growing number of civil legal cases that involve health care practitioners, e.g., health care malpractice. It is important to be aware of both civil and criminal legal systems and the impact they may have on your practice (Scott, 1997).

Laws tell us what we shouldn't do, and are based on formal rules that if violated are subject to legal sanctions. Ethics give us standards to live by and guide our professional conduct. Sanctions for violating ethical codes are administered by professional associations (Scott, 1997).

Major Ethical Theories

Theories provide a way to look at ethical issues and help us decide which course of action to take. There are many ethical theories, but you will probably hear predominately two major categories discussed; *teleology* and *deontology*. It is also not uncommon to hear people use a blend of these theories when making decisions about health care. A strict teleological point of view may not always be acceptable because of its lack of respect for individual autonomy, whereas a strict deontological approach may not be totally acceptable because of its reliance on acts of duty. It is important that you understand your own philosophical views when discussing ethical issues with others.

Teleological Theory (Utilitarianism)

When people make decisions based on this theory, they are most likely to decide based on the consequences of the act. The word teleology comes from the Greek *telos* which means "the end" The goal of teleological theory is to do good and avoid harm. The major principle for resolving ethical conflicts is to produce the greatest balance of good over bad or to produce the greatest good for the greatest number. The worth of an action is judged by the consequences, thus the goal of the action or "end" (result) justifies the means.

Deontological Theory

The theory of deontology emphasizes identification of what your duty is, and the major goal is to respect others. The word *deon* is Greek for "duty". This philosophy states that the act itself, or the means, is what is important, not always the consequence. Deontologists resolve ethical conflicts by weighing conflicting duties to various individuals to determine which is the primary or actual duty (Graber, 1988).

Moral Development

In the 1950s, Lawrence Kohlberg conducted studies that identified three levels of moral development (Kohlberg, 1984). These levels represent the reasons that people have for choosing certain moral actions. Because the focus of this theory is on cognition and the sequential stages of moral reasoning, it is called cognitive-developmental theory. In the first level, the pre-conventional level, people respond to what is right and wrong and are essentially driven by consequences of behavior so as to avoid punishment or obtain rewards. At the conventional level, people choose to be right in order to avoid the disapproval of others and to conform to the rules of society (laws). In the third, post-conventional level, people make choices based on their own personal values and principles. At this level they are concerned with public welfare and universal principles of justice. Development through these levels is a gradual process and may cease at any stage (Kohlberg, 1984).

Kohlberg found that moral development varies from person to person and is not a function of age. In fact, much of the applied ethics research shows that the most influential factor on the level of moral reasoning is the number of years of formal education. It is thought that more years of education expose a person to diverse ways of looking at the world and solving problems, and consequently increase levels of moral reasoning. Rest (1994) hypothesizes that the reason for this is that individuals who go on to higher education love to learn, enjoy intellectual stimulation, are more involved in their communities, and take more interest in larger societal issues. This does not mean that a person reasoning at a higher moral level has more intelligence, rather it means that these individuals have better conceptual tools for making sense out of the world and for decision-making. These individuals are able to think more critically and see what might be best for individuals and society as a whole (Rest, 1994).

James Rest built upon and expanded Kohlberg's theory and developed what he calls the *four-component model* (Rest, 1979). He says that there is more to moral reasoning than cognition and identifies four psychological components which he thinks determine moral behavior. These are moral sensitivity (interpreting the situation), moral judgment (judging which action is morally right or wrong), moral motivation (prioritizing moral values relative to other values), and moral character (having courage, persistence, and implementing skills to act morally) (Rest, 1994).

Ethical Problem-Solving

We do not have to be ethical experts to be involved in the process of ethical reasoning. Knowing the basic principles and understanding your own professional code of ethics provides a foundation. Many processes for ethical decision-making have been put forward, most of which are representative of typical problem-solving techniques. It is important, as a first step, to examine the facts in the particular situation that you view as an ethical dilemma. Be sure you have collected all relevant facts and check the reliability of these facts. Second, you must identify what makes this an ethical problem. What are the moral issues or principles involved and what foreseeable consequences might come of this situation? Third, you must engage in a process of weighing the moral issues and ethical principles as they relate to potential consequences. What is most important? Fourth, identify the options available to you to act ethically according to your own reasoning about what is right and wrong. And finally, select one of the options based on ethical guidelines as well as any relevant legal implications. Acting on your decision can often be the hardest part and requires that you be strong and clear in your reasons for action. In ethics, good intentions do not always bring good deeds. It is important that you implement your ethical decision.

Developing Professionalism

The development of professional behaviors is much more than just good health care manners or etiquette. Being dependable, presenting oneself professionally, showing initiative, being empathetic, cooperating with other team members, being organized, using clinical reasoning, giving and receiving constructive feedback, and demonstrating clear verbal and written communication are all professional behaviors that can be developed and learned. Professional behaviors link back to ethics because they are the ways in which we, as health care practitioners, can demonstrate our concern and caring for others in society.

Dependability is grounded in the ethical principles of beneficence and fidelity. Being late for therapy sessions or meetings can negatively impact our goal as health care professionals to provide useful and effective services for our clients or maintain good working relationships with team members. Fidelity means that we keep our promises and meet the expectations of our clients, as well as being competent in what we do.

Professional presentation of oneself and communicating interest and a positive attitude toward our clients and coworkers tells them that we care about our relationships and the well-being of those to whom we provide services. A professional and positive attitude can give our clients a sense of trust in our competence to provide services that will benefit them. The professional behavior of demonstrating initiative also is grounded in the ethical principles of beneficence and our concern for doing the best job that we can for our clients.

Empathy is a key professional behavior that demonstrates our concern for others and a respect for the ideas and opinions of others when making ethical decisions about health care. Cooperation with other health care practitioners demonstrates a respect for their autonomy and leads to better outcomes for our clients.

Clinical reasoning is a professional behavior that is needed to solve ethical dilemmas. The ethical reasoning process and problem-solving ethical dilemmas require that you be able to gather and interpret information, analyze information, as well as generate potential solutions to the situation.

The professional behaviors of verbal communication, written communication, and supervisory process relate to the ethical principles of veracity, fidelity, confidentiality and privacy. All of these principles serve to create and sustain trusting relationships with clients and co-workers.

Concluding Remarks

Ethics and values will form the base for your development as a professional. Understanding and developing your own personal morals and principles will help you to identify ethical dilemmas and make good decisions for your clients and patients. Professional behaviors are the vehicle through which you act upon or implement your ethical principles. These professional behaviors can be learned and developed as you become socialized into your respective professions and will help you when you need to take those tough ethical stances.

References

American Nurses Association (1985). *Professional code of ethics for nurses.* Kansas City, MO: Author.

Beauchamp, T. L. & Childress, J. F. (1994). *Principles of Biomedical Ethics,* Third Edition. New York, NY: Oxford University Press.

Brody, H. (1994). *Framing the health reform debate.* Hastings Center Report, May-June, 7-8

Craven, R. & Hirnle (1996). Ethical and legal concerns. In R. Craven & Hirnle, *Fundamentals of Nursing,* Second Edition, (pp. 38-61). Philadelphia, PA: Lippincott-Raven.

Graber, G. C., (1988). Basic theories in medical ethics. In J. F. Monagle & D. C. Thomasma (Eds.), *Medical ethics: a guide for health professionals* (pp. 462-475). Rockville, MD: Aspen.

Hansen, R. (1998). Ethics in occupational therapy. In M. E. Neistadt & E. B. Crepeau (Eds.), *Willard & Spackman's Occupational Therapy,* (pp. 819-827). Philadelphia, PA: Lippincott.

Kohlberg, L. (1984). *Essays on moral development, volume II: The psychology of moral development.* San Francisco, CA: Harper & Row.

Mosey, A. C. (1992). *Applied scientific inquiry in the health professions: an epistemological orientation.* Rockville, MD: AOTA.

Opacich, K. J. (1996). Ethical dimensions in occupational therapy. In J. Bair & M. Gray (Eds.), *The Occupational Therapy Manager,* (pp.627-650). Bethesda, MD: The American Occupational Therapy Association.

Purtillo, R. (1993). *Ethical dimensions in the health professions,* Second edition. Philadelphia, PA: W.B. Saunders.

Purtillo, R. & Haddad, A. (1996). *Health professional and patient interaction.* Philadelphia, PA: W.B. Saunders.

Rest, J. R. (1979). *Development in judging moral issues.* Minneapolis, MN: University of Minnesota Press.

Rest, J. R. (1994). Background: Theory and research. In J.R. Rest & D. Narvaez (Eds.), *Moral development in the professions* (pp. 1-26). Hillsdale, NJ: Erlbaum.

Scott, R. (1997). *Promoting legal awareness in physical and occupational therapy.* St. Louis, MO: Mosby.

Sieghart, P. (1985). Professions as the conscience of society. *Journal of Medical Ethics, 11,* 117-122.

Tourigny, A. (1992). Why professional associations have codes of ethics. *OT Week,* November, 6-7.

Veatch, R. M. & Flack, H. E. (1997). *Case studies in allied health ethics.* Upper Saddle River, NJ: Prentice Hall.

Chapter Three

Developmental Framework

Mary E. Muscari, PhD, CRNP, CS

A seasoned practitioner assists a student in treating the burned hands of an 8-year-old boy. During the painful procedure, the wide-eyed boy stiffens and declares, "I won't cry. I'm real tough."

"You sure are brave," says the student.

The practitioner looks into the boy's eyes and quietly whispers, "It's okay to cry."

The boy's eyes fill with tears.

What did the seasoned practitioner know that the student did not, and why?

The practitioner quickly analyzed and interpreted the child's cues by using knowledge of child development and nonverbal communication. School-age children can react to hospitalization and illness with the underlying defense mechanism of reaction formation. The boy said he was tough when he actually was very frightened. His rigid and wide-eyed appearance signaled fear. The student may have had the necessary knowledge, but most likely lacked the analytical ability to quickly interpret the situation while simultaneously preparing for a procedure. Clinical reasoning is a professional behavior that develops with time and experience.

Professional behaviors are not innate, they must be cultivated and carefully nurtured through their natural developmental process. Today's student matures into tomorrow's seasoned professional.

Professional behaviors are needed to provide quality client service, effectively market oneself, conduct research, and keep pace with the legal, political, ethical, social, and economic environments. The term professionalism lacks uniformity in both its definition and interpretation. Criteria include intensive, extended education and preceptorship (Fidler, 1979); an organized and specialized body of knowledge; an ability to gain society's trust; autonomy; a code of ethics; and the assumption of responsibility, accountability, and liability (Breines, 1988). Professionals are viewed as leaders in specialized areas who make sound decisions and contribute expert opinions (Adams, Miller & Beck, 1996). They are problem-solvers who analyze client needs, demonstrate accountability and responsibility, pursue consultation, communicate and work effectively with peers and other disciplines (Gandy & Jensen, 1992).

Thus, professionalism requires specific knowledge, attitudes, and values, all of which are exemplified by professional behaviors. These behaviors are dependability, professional presentation, initiative, empathy, cooperation, organization, clinical reasoning, supervisory process, verbal communication, and written communication (Kasar, Clark, Watson, & Pfister, 1996) (Table 3-1). However, it is virtually impossible for any individual to begin a career with such a repertoire of characteristics and abilities. Professional behaviors must be developed and enhanced in students and clinicians throughout their entire developmental process.

The professional behavior developmental process can be best delineated using an Erikson framework to demonstrate stages, growth patterns, and potential problems (Edelman & Mandle, 1994; Erikson, 1993; Schuster & Ashburn, 1992). As with Erikson's original Eight Stages of

Table 3-1

PROFESSIONAL BEHAVIORS

DEPENDABILITY

Completing tasks on schedule
Ensuring cost-effective health care
Complying with expanding accountability
Providing accessible care within the emerging health care
   system

PROFESSIONAL PRESENTATION

Presenting oneself in a manner acceptable to clients, peers
   and colleagues
Using body posture and affect to communicate interest or
   engaged attention
Conveying positive attitude toward role
Enhancing visibility of role

INITIATIVE

Demonstrating energetic, positive, motivated manner
Self-starting projects, tasks and programs
Taking initiative to direct own continuous learning
Demonstrating change agent skills

EMPATHY

Being sensitive and responding to the feelings and
   behaviors of others
Listening to and considering the ideas and opinions of others
Responding with sensitivity to the needs of other profes-
   sionals
Rendering assistance to all individuals without bias

COOPERATION

Involving clients and families in the decision-making
   process
Working effectively with others
Developing group cohesiveness by assisting in their
   development
Becoming an active member of regional, state and/or
   national groups

ORGANIZATION

Prioritizing self and tasks
Managing time to meet client and organizational requirements
Using organization skills to contribute to the development of others

CLINICAL REASONING

Analyzing, synthesizing, and interpreting information
Giving alternative solutions to complex issues and situations
Utilizing, evaluating, and conducting research
Demonstrating ethical decision-making skills

SUPERVISORY PROCESS

Modifying performance in response to meaningful feedback
Operating within the scope of one's own skills and seeking assistance when needed
Demonstrating clinical and professional leadership
Utilizing consultation, collaboration, and referral skills
   appropriately

VERBAL COMMUNICATION

Sharing perceptions and opinions with clarity and quality
   of content
Verbalizing opposing opinions with constructive results
Utilizing teaching skills for clients, students, peers, and
   colleagues
Making formal presentations at regional, state, and/or
   national conferences

WRITTEN COMMUNICATION

Communicating ideas and opinions clearly and concisely
   in written reports
Writing research reports
Writing for publication

Adapted from Kasar, Clark, Watson, & Pfister (1996). Professional Development Assessment. Unpublished form.

Man, students and clinicians undergo a series of crises — conflicts between two opposing forces — that must be dealt with by using maturational experiences. These crises evolve over time, require changes in behaviors and thinking, and occasionally create feelings of unbalance. Students and clinicians must successfully complete each stage of professional development to move to the next. Failure to successfully complete a stage may result in the person becoming stuck in that stage and unable to progress.

Benner's (1984) model of expert performance is also used to depict the progression of experience from novice to expert. This transition requires long and steady practice, sustained motivation, and the efficiency of strategies based on organizing, storing, and utilizing knowledge. The model of professional practice facilitates the transition from novice to expert. This framework varies by using only three levels, novice, apprentice, and expert, each containing appropriate stages (Table 3-2).

Table 3-2

PROFESSIONAL BEHAVIOR LEVELS AND STAGES

LEVELS	STAGES
NOVICE	Trust vs. Mistrust
	Autonomy vs. Shame and Doubt
	Intimacy vs. Guilt
APPRENTICE	Industry vs. Inferiority
	Identity vs. Role Confusion
	Intimacy vs. Isolation
EXPERT	Generativity vs. Stagnation
	Integrity vs. Despair

Students and clinicians must continuously strive to enhance their professionalism through education and practice, and educators and supervisors must continuously promote professional behavior development through modeling, mentoring, and the provision of evaluative feedback.

Novice

Beginning novices have no experience in the tasks that they need to perform, and are given situations in terms of objective attributes such as measurements and deadlines. Rules must be followed and behaviors are extremely limited and inflexible. Unfortunately, rules cannot convey all professional behaviors. They can teach a student to hand in reports when due, however, rules cannot develop empathy, motivation, or cooperation. These and other traits must develop and mature throughout the developmental process.

Advanced beginners have coped with real situations enough to learn their aspects. Aspects are global characteristics that can be learned only through experience. For example, the ability to communicate complex subject matter depends on the new graduate's previous experience with that subject matter. Advanced beginners devise principles that dictate actions in terms of both attributes and aspects, and they need to spend a great deal of time on aspect recognition.

Stage 1 — Trust Vs. Mistrust

In this stage, the student enters the professional arena as a *blank slate* whose significant other is the educator. The central focus is the development of a sense of trust in educators and the new professional environment. This sense of trust forms the foundation for all future professional behaviors. The quality of the educator/student relationship is a critical element in the development of trust. Students who receive attentive care learn that they can be assisted in having their educational needs met. In turn, these students begin to demonstrate the onset of professional behaviors, such as being on time and having an energetic manner.

In contrast, students experiencing consistently delayed or unmet needs develop a sense of uncertainty, leading to the mistrust of educators and the environment. Students may become suspicious of others in their educational environment, crippling their ability to progress in their professional development. These students may demonstrate negative behaviors, such as tardiness and lack of motivation.

A significant accomplishment in this stage is the answering of the question, "Is this what I really want to be when I grow up?" Most students enter professional programs knowing their goals. They have a strong desire to help others and to learn and perform the various roles of their chosen discipline. However, there are those who are not so certain. Some students enter a discipline to please their parents, some to attain employment or salary opportunities, and others to compensate for an inability to enter their true chosen field. If the answer to the question is an affirmative "yes," then students begin to learn to trust their own instincts. However, if the answer is negative or ambivalent, students immediately mistrust their instincts. The student becomes stuck in this stage, paving the way for possible failure in professional development.

The crisis of trust vs. mistrust is not totally resolved during the early educational experience. It arises again with each phase of professional development and with each significant situational crisis. For example, a seasoned professional may experience a "mid-career crisis," or an extremely difficult client or administrative problem causing that professional to question himself, "Is this what I *really* want to do with my life?" The resulting answers are the same, thus, both trust and mistrust may be reinforced or converted throughout the development process.

Stage 2 — Autonomy Vs. Shame and Doubt

Once students develop a sense of trust, they are ready to give up dependence in order to assert their blooming sense of control, independence, and autonomy. They begin to master individuation (differentiation of self from other students), separation from educator(s), control over basic skills, communication with new terminology, acquisition of professionally acceptable behavior, and early interactions with established professionals in the clinical arena. The student has learned that his or her educators are predictable and reliable; now the student begins to learn that his or her own behavior has a predictable, reliable effect on others. The student is more capable of meeting self-learning needs and begins to assert independence.

Students' developing skills become the means for the development of professional self-concept and self-esteem. They take pride in their accomplishments, want to do everything independently, and challenge their educators with their new found ability to say "no," to test the limits of their own power. The struggling student who really wants and needs assistance may initially refuse it just to express autonomy. These abilities allow for more professional awareness as students scrutinize their new found self-concept over and over again. Students repeatedly test their newly learned language (discipline-related terminology) and motor skills (assessment and intervention techniques) on family and friends who may be alternately supportive and frustrated at the students' eagerness and persistence. Here is where students realize that family and friends really do not understand what they are going through, an awareness that forms better peer alliance, more cooperation, and greater empathy.

Students should explore their new found skills with both vigor and restraint. They need to be zealous in their desire to perform well, yet tempered to take the time to learn the principles behind their skills and the lessons of their mistakes. Growing professionals must walk before they run — but on their own two feet.

A sense of shame and doubt can develop if students are kept dependent in areas where they are capable of using newly acquired skills, or if they are made to feel inadequate when attempting new skills. Students often continue to seek a familiar security object, such as a previously accomplished skill (vital sign monitoring, neurological assessment) or prior knowledge learned from non-professional experience ("When my Uncle Joe had emphysema..."), during times of stress. These should be viewed as temporary and common lapses, and the student should be encouraged to examine the stressor for problem-solving. Unfortunately, when students do fail to develop a sense of autonomy, they learn to doubt their abilities and refrain from trying. Such a student may continuously lag behind peers in later stages or even fail out of the program.

Stage 3 — Initiative Vs. Guilt

New graduate professionals continue to develop their sense of self-concept through task- and career-oriented skills. Success builds self-esteem, and career acceptance reinforces their roles as professionals. Professional roles are explored through their ability to ask "why" questions and seek new explanations as reality and theory begin to clash.

By this stage, new graduates normally master a sense of autonomy and move on to master a sense of initiative. The new graduate is an energetic, enthusiastic, and sometimes intrusive learner with idealistic vision. Professional conscience (the inner voice that responds to situations involving professional choices) begins to develop. New graduates explore the professional world with all of their senses and powers, relying on repetition to develop mastery. They also want to be a helpful member of the team. Unfortunately, their lack of experience and entry-level organizational skills may sometimes make them more of a hindrance than a help, resulting in failure and chaos. Sensitive supervisors realize that the intent is just as important as the task. They encourage new graduates to keep trying and to enhance their skills through inservice programs, continuing education, and the mentoring process. Professional new graduates then eagerly receive the constructive criticism and modify their performance according to the meaningful feedback. Professionals always know to operate within the scope of their own practice and to seek guidance when needed.

Development of a sense of guilt occurs when the new graduate is made to feel that his or her idealism and activities are unacceptable. Guilt, anxiety, and fear result when the new graduate's thoughts and activities clash with colleague and supervisor expectations. Guilt may also arise if new graduates are unable to live up to their own expectations. The transition from student to clinician is an extremely challenging experience as expectations and workload increase and one-to-one support decreases. New graduates must learn to set realistic goals for themselves, realizing that, although advanced, they are still beginners.

Apprentice

Professionals who face the same situations for 2 to 3 years typically demonstrate competence. Competence develops when clinicians see their actions in terms of long-term goals. Plans are based on considerable conscious, abstract, analytical contemplation of the problem. Competent clinicians lack the speed and flexibility of the proficient professional, however, they have a feeling of mastery and the ability to manage many clinical contingencies.

Competence still prevails with the deliberate planning that is characteristic of this level. There is efficiency and organization after what seems to be great effort. Competence can be enhanced by planning and coordinating care for more complex clients, which enables the clinician to move toward proficiency.

The proficient clinician is the one who most frequently notes deterioration or client problems prior to explicit changes. This is the clinician who has worked with the same population for 3 to 5 years and who regresses to the competent level when faced with novelty or the demand for an analytic, procedural description.

Stage 4 — Industry Vs. Inferiority

The clinician normally completes the first three developmental tasks and focuses on mastering industry. A feel of industry grows out of a desire for real achievement. Clinicians engage in tasks and activities that they can carry through to completion. They learn rules, how to compete with others, and how to cooperate to achieve goals. Professional and social peer relationships become increasingly important sources of support. Listening abilities are enhanced and the clinician shows more consideration for the group. Teamwork is a medium for achieving shared goals in providing client service.

Increasing cognitive and motor skills, peer persuasion, and greater professional awareness all influence the clinician's self-concept, which includes self-esteem, a sense of control, and role. However, self-esteem is still based in the core peer group, and clinicians need to know that they are appreciated for who they are and what they do. Clinicians with positive self-esteem see themselves as capable, significant, worthy, and successful. Those with a sense of control are able to make choices and feel in charge of themselves. Clinicians with an internal locus of control feel responsible for themselves and their actions, and tend to achieve at higher levels than those with an external locus of control. The latter group feels that their actions are controlled by others or fate, leaving them with a sense of powerlessness. Clinicians who understand their professional role(s) are more apt to fulfill them than those who lack that understanding. Success or failure with peers beyond the core group greatly influences their self-concept, and new clinicians need time to develop their own unique interests. As they move through this stage, the opinions of supervisors also become critical forces in self-esteem development. Maturation also brings a sense of control over the professional self and environment.

Clinicians can develop a sense of inferiority stemming from unrealistic expectations or a sense of failing to meet standards set for them by others. Because they feel inadequate, self-esteem sags. There is an inability to take pride in one's work, which could result in stagnation of professional behaviors. It is difficult to demonstrate initiative and a positive attitude with low self-esteem.

Stage 5 — Identity Vs. Role Confusion

Once clinicians have progressed past the beginning stage, they begin to form a greater sense of professional identity by integrating everything they have learned into a whole to learn who they are and where they fit in. Clinicians further develop a professional self-concept through identity formation, relying on peers for acceptance. Anything that is viewed as a defect is magnified and becomes the focus for intense examination. Negative views of defects, either real or perceived, can result in serious damage to self-perception and self-concept. As they grow professionally, clinicians become more capable of internalizing positive self-perceptions, viewing the competencies and values that will continue throughout their career.

The radius of significant others is the peer group. Cohesiveness is better evolved. Development of who he or she is and where he or she is going becomes a central focus. The clinician continues to redefine his or her self-concept and roles that he or she can play with certainty. As changes occur, he or she must reintegrate the previous trust in their abilities, themselves, and how they appear to others.

Identity formation is stressful and difficult work. The clinician looks not only to peers and immediate colleagues, but also to professional organizations. These organizations may vary in complexity, philosophy, and subspecialty (e.g., American Occupational Therapy Association [AOTA], American Nurses' Association [ANA], Sensory Integration International [SII], Association of Certified Hand Therapists [ACHT], National Association of Pediatric Nurse Associates and Practitioners [NAPNAP], and state and local groups). Clinicians can easily face role confusion as they try to focus their identity in one or more areas. The clinician's professional identity is also influenced by the extent to which earlier tasks were completed. Those who experienced earlier successes are likely to form solvent professional identities. Resourceful clinicians can develop strong identities even if they encountered some earlier failures. However, persistent failure is likely to result in lack of professional identity and a sense of role confusion.

The inability to develop a sense of who he or she is and what he or she can become results in role diffusion and an inability to solve core conflicts. It is probably at this point that some professionals develop a sense of career apathy, resulting in deteriorating professional behaviors or leaving their careers all together.

Stage 6 — Intimacy Vs. Isolation

Once clinicians establish a sense of personal professional identity they are able to develop greater relationships with colleagues and other disciplines without losing that self-identity. In the early part of this stage, clinicians may become fearful of losing their identity, especially those in professions whose knowledge and skills overlap with other disciplines. Intimacy involves more contact, so clinicians must be more interactive with one another, both on the job and off. The work environment is insufficient in creating a sense of intimacy. The hectic pace allows little time for professional interaction, let alone the intimacy of discussion and sharing. Professional development requires active participation in professional groups regardless of level or specialty. Here, clinicians engage in

the sharing of knowledge as well as perceptions, opinions and experiences, creating mutual satisfaction and support, and adding further competence to allow the clinician to reach the level of proficiency.

Intimacy avoidance leads to professional isolation. The clinician feels alone and detached. Career goals are lost and professional behaviors lag far behind those of colleagues. The clinician may also develop faulty attachments, especially if identity formation is poor. This clinician may attempt to identify with professionals from another field, further blurring his or her professional self-concept. Professional relationships with other disciplines are necessary; however, boundaries should be identified and respected.

Expert

Expert performers no longer rely on analytic principles to connect situations to actions. Due to enormous experiential backgrounds, experts have an intuitive grasp of situations and the ability to hone in on problems without wasting time. However, expertise is not always descriptive because the expert operates from a deep understanding of total situations. Comments may be as nondescript as, "It doesn't feel right" or "I just know it." Experts may also respond to hypothetical questions with responses such as, "It all depends."

Expert clinicians can also provide consultative services for other clinicians, both in and outside their disciplines. They are very effective in detecting early changes and making recommendations. In the past, many experts had little opportunity to compare and develop consensus on their observations. Now with the advent of the Internet and servers, experts are free to network around the world.

Stage 7 — Generativity Vs. Stagnation

Now it is the clinician's turn to contribute to the next generation of budding professionals.

There is a feeling of productivity and creativity evidenced by reaching one's professional goals. Proficient professionals become expert and share that expertise with others. They are motivated to develop and nurture young professionals, and to leave their mark on the world. Generativity means passing on one's legacy and knowledge, thus leaving one's mark. This can be accomplished by precepting students, orienting new graduates, teaching in the academic setting, presenting at conferences, conducting research or writing articles. All of these require a level of expertise and fulfill the desire to be needed.

Lack of accomplishment results in professional stagnation. The clinician feels a sense of boredom and emptiness that may result in self-absorption. This clinician is frustrated just by the thought of contribution and becomes the negative role model easily agitated by the eager student or new graduate. This clinician never reaches the level of professional expert, regardless of knowledge and skill capacity, due to the lack of many of the other professional behaviors.

This is also the stage of critical self-review, and even the most competent clinicians can be disappointed in themselves and their accomplishments. Personal and professional values undergo both major and minor changes as patterns are set. Clinicians now move in a number of directions as many of the goals of major institutions are created by persons in this reflective stage. They may become more politically active in either their professional organization or in government matters related to health care. They may advance in the administrative or educational arenas, or they may grow as researchers or writers. Many return to school to seek advanced degrees, some in advanced practice. There are also those who feel that they have met all their desired professional goals and decide to move on to another career. Regardless of the choice, at this stage all clinicians explore the meaning of their career by reevaluating choices, purposes, and the expenditure of resources. It is a period of reservation as well as opportunity.

Stage 8 — Integrity Vs. Despair

Integrity signifies the way one has lived and is still living his or her professional life. It is the subjective realization that the choices and decisions made in various life stages were the best ones possible at those times, and it is the evaluation that one is still in control of one's professional life. Just as the student learned trust as successful completion of the first stage, the expert learns that satisfactory retirement is successful completion of the final stage. Integrity provides the experience that retirement is the resolution of a successful career.

Failure to master integrity results in despair. This is a state of conflict over the way one has lived and continues to live his or her professional life. It is the subjective experience of dissatisfaction, disgust, or disappointment accompanied by the feeling that things would have been done differently if given the chance. There is a feeling of anxiety over the future and a sense of lack of control. The reality of retirement becomes a source of fear.

Successful completion of this stage also relies on successful completion of all the previous ones. Those clinicians who have difficulty at this stage, probably had difficulty in earlier ones. The opposite is also true. However, there are always those who, despite earlier success, struggle in the final stage; and those who, despite previous failures, become successful in later life. This certainly demonstrates that persons can adjust their professional development throughout their lifespan.

Looking into the Future

Professionals are perceived as leaders in specialized areas who make sound decisions and contribute expert opinions (Adams, Miller & Beck, 1996). They are the problem solvers who demonstrate accountability and responsibility, analyze clients' needs, communicate effectively, pursue consultation, and work effectively with other disciplines (Gandy & Jensen, 1992). Professionals also demonstrate initiative, empathy, dependability, and organizational skills.

Today's health care professionals are expected to exemplify these behaviors and more.

References

Adams, D., Miller, B., & Beck, L. (1996). Professionalism behaviors of hospital nurse executives and middle managers in 10 western states. *Western Journal of Nursing Research, 18(1)*, 77-88.

Benner, P. (1984). *From novice to expert.* Melona Park, CA: Addison-Wesley Publishing Co.

Breines, E. (1988). Redefining professionalism for occupational therapy. *The American Journal of Occupational Therapy, 42,* 55-57.

Erikson, E. (1993). *Childhood and society.* New York, NY: WW Norton.

Fidler, G. (1979). Professional or nonprofessional. *Occupational Therapy: 2001 AD.* (pp 31-36). Rockville, MD: AOTA.

Gandy, J., & Jensen, G. (1992). Group work and reflective practicums in physical therapy education: Models for professional behavior development. *Journal of Physical Therapy Education, 6(1),* 6-10.

Kasar, J., Clark, E. N., Watson., D., & Pfister, S. (1996). *Professional Development Assessment.* Unpublished form.

Schuster, C., & Ashburn, S. (1992). *The process of human development,* Third Edition. Philadelphia, PA: JB Lippincott.

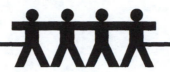

Part Two

The Right Stuff: Professional Behaviors

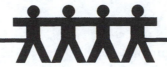

Chapter Four

Dependability

Paul Petersen,
PhD, OTR/L

Dependability Defined

From the Dictionary

For over 4 months, writer William Ecenbarger traveled through 28 states displaying both his teeth and a set of recent X-rays to 50 randomly selected dentists. He sought estimates for the dental work needed, and he discussed his situation with each dentist. The family was relocating to the area for a new job, he explained. Recent gum surgery was successful, and he was seeking a new dentist. He added that his employer had a direct pay dental plan where the dentist merely submitted the bill for reimbursement. This plan is attractive as payment is fast, and there is no third party such as an insurance company to question the work.

Prior to his trip, Ecenbarger discussed his dental work with his dentist of 15 years. He needed a crown on tooth number 30, and the cost would be less than $500. He then saw three other dentists whom he trusted. They were recognized in the field and had no financial interest in his case. Among them they agreed that the crown for No. 30 was the only immediate problem. But they added that No. 18 might need a crown or filling in the future. He should have to pay no more than $1500, they told him, even if two crowns were recommended. These estimates were his base for comparison as he traveled around the country. In a special report to the *Reader's Digest*, Ecenbarger (1997) disclosed his findings. What did he learn? The estimates he received for his dental work ranged from under $500 to as high as $29,850! Equally as startling was that 15 of the 50 examining dentists missed the problem in tooth No. 30 entirely.

Throughout this chapter the topic of dependability will be used in close association with reliability and personal responsibility. While there is overlap among the terms, as they are used interchangeably in some literature, small distinctions remain. Dependability cannot be studied outside of responsibility and reliability. This chapter will convey the spirit of how a dependable and reliable health care practitioner should behave in order to develop a sense of trust in the clinical arena.

In the *Random House Unabridged Dictionary*, "dependable" is defined as worthy of trust, reliable, and capable of being depended upon. In the same volume, the definition of "reliable" denotes that a person may be relied on, dependable in achievement, and honest. "Responsible" means answerable, accountable within one's power, having capacity for moral decisions, and capable of rational thought or action. *Webster's Third New International Dictionary* (unabridged) contains similar definitions of dependability and reliability to those in Random House, but to "responsible" it adds morally, legally, or mentally accountable, related to trustworthiness, and of decent appearance.

From an engineering perspective, Kececiogly (1991) characterizes reliability as the probability that a system or its parts will perform what they were intended to do within a given level of confidence. Husted (1993) applies reliability to organizational development and views it as consistency of a procedure, design, or system to produce the same results. Conceptualized, reliability stands for the organization's tolerance for failure. Reliability becomes a tool of organizational design, with the goal of making ethical decisions. Ethical failure, then, is a form of system breakdown. Husted (1993) reminds us of familiar reliability breakdowns, including the catastrophic toxin release in Bhopal, India, and Alaska's *Exxon Valdez* oil tanker spill.

From the Clinic

While preparing this chapter, I conducted an informal survey of my patients to see how the above definitions applied in a small clinical sample. Patients were from an outpatient clinic, and a majority of them had work-related injuries. Some of these patients were asked directly for their opinions regarding important qualities of health care providers. Others let their opinions be known throughout the course of their treatment.

This is a synopsis of what was heard: "...Is a good listener, takes the time needed and does not rush me, a therapist (nurse, physician, etc,) I feel I can trust, does not keep me waiting too long, knows his or her stuff, friendly, respects me as a person, refers me to someone else if necessary, is usually accessible, timely and accurate with paperwork, calls me back, flexible, bonds with me, answers my questions, does not overcharge, pays attention to details, shares information with colleagues about me as needed, puts my child (or me) first, is open to alternative approaches, truly cares about me, takes my feelings and ideas (preferences) into consideration, and is passionate about what he or she does." It is obvious that medical and technical expertise is a given assumption for these patients. Their concern, instead, is directed to their practitioner's supportive behaviors which define dependability and other topics in this text.

The patients' responses reinforced the TV news coverage citing that Americans have definite health needs that are highly personal and of great importance. They take a risk when they put their care in our hands. They want help that is competent and efficient. Most of all, they want providers they can trust. The average person on the street is open but naive when approaching all providers as equally skilled and trustworthy. It is an unsatisfactory personal experience with a provider that will change his or her mind.

Significance

Importance of Dependability

When asked to contribute the chapter on dependability for this text, I was in the process of writing a letter to the editor of our local newspaper about the topic to express my frustration and exasperation. There were errors in our insurance policies (car, life, home, and health!), retirement computation, tree service, lawn service, magazine subscriptions, mail orders (mistakes made in both our and their favor), miscellaneous billing problems, car servicing difficulties, and more. Some contractors never showed up to complete their contract or did marginal work. Some goods we purchased did not work, were broken, or had parts missing. The list goes on.

These disappointments took considerable time to straighten out with calls, return visits, letters, mailings, faxes, and requests to send in duplicate paperwork. Every adjustment required several steps, passing through numerous clerks, representatives, or voice mail. Each promised complete satisfaction. Problems in dependability appear to be epidemic.

DEPENDABILITY AND THE GENERAL CONSUMER POPULATION

The lack of dependability can have more serious consequences than one's lost time or irritation. Examples were recently reported in our local newspaper and television news. An elderly customer's electric power was shut off for billing errors, a plant superintendent received the wrong parts shipment for an important production deadline, and a car was unable to stop following a recent brake repair. In health care, these deficiencies are costly for the patient and provider alike, resulting in prolonged illness, legal action, and in some cases, death. One needs only to recall the pattern of incidents in a Florida hospital where the wrong limb was amputated.

Health care is portrayed by the media in endless polls that typically cover politicians, the economy, and the readiness of the computer chip for the turn of the millennium. Is the level of trust, or lack of trust, in health care on a par with that for politicians, lobbyists, and special interest groups? If all was well in the health care arena, the polls addressing satisfaction levels with providers, insurance plans, HMOs, and institutions would not be on television. Good health rarely makes the news unless it is sensational, such as the recent transplantation of a cadaver arm to a long-term amputee.

We know from the polls that a portion of consumers are dissatisfied with all or parts of their health care. Why are they losing confidence, and what can we do about it? Despite our country's high ranking in health care delivery, there is certainly room for improvement. Many mistakenly think that legislation, regulation, and higher taxes can resolve these problems. While the faceless "institution" is under fire, it must be remembered that a resurgence in consumer confidence begins with dedicated individuals exerting leadership to provide a commitment to the best care for their patients (Souba, 1996).

DEPENDABILITY AS TRUST

Beyond "doing no harm" in the professional sense, one of the greatest goals for providers is to establish trust in relationships with patients. While this book and chapter are not entitled "trust", developing trust is essentially what this book is about. It is our initiative, our empathy, our cooperation, our organization, and our communication that define the level of trust our patients have for us. Trust becomes the catalyst that maximizes the efficacy of the services we deliver.

Trust is the reason one's choice of health care practitioner is so sacred to the American public. Addressing the leadership of academic medical centers, Souba (1996) remarked that it is trust, direction, and hope that are expected of leaders in the profession. Trust is the most important factor of the health care leader's success. Trust is called for outside of health care. Consider research conducted in the business world in Moorman, Deshpande, and Zaltman's (1993) multivariate study on factors influencing trust in market research. They found that integrity, confidentiality, expertise, demonstrated sincerity, and timeliness were some of the more important variables that contributed to the development of trust in the marketing relationships studied.

Reconsider the nightly TV media polls. These polls are asking Americans about their level of confidence or trust in their physicians, politicians, and/or their readiness for the coming millennium. When trust is lacking, effectiveness fails, so it is important that we consider ways to build trust. This is best summed up in a quotation by Booker T. Washington, "Few things help an individual more than to place responsibility on him, and to let him know that you trust him" (Coy, 1985, p. 328).

INDIVIDUAL VS. CORPORATE RESPONSIBILITY

While this chapter emphasizes dependability and personal responsibility, there is a higher level that we are all a part of, which is institutional responsibility. Institution denotes an established society, a corporate body created for the purpose of promoting a particular objective. Examples include organizations such as a hospital, health care alliance, university, or professional society.

A few years ago Souba (1996, citing Bellah, et al.) addressed the role of institutional responsibility. It is, after all, the institution that provides the necessary context within which we become individuals. It both enables and restrains us, and provides us with the environments and conditions where our character is tested and formed. "This is in part because some of our institutions have indeed grown out of control and beyond our comprehension. But the answer is to change them, for it is illusory to think that we can escape them" (p. 7).

Let us consider institutional responsibility in relation to the opening scenario of this chapter, the one where Ecenbarger (1997) received a variety of diagnoses, care plans, and cost estimates for his dental work. Dental leaders responded immediately to his story. While some individuals expressed concern for the reported observations, others attacked *Reader's Digest*, the methodology, or simply provided damage control or "spin".

The editor of the *Journal of the American Dental Association* found Ecenbarger's (1997) article to be a bashing of the dental profession. He said it was *Reader's Digest's* "desire to generate controversy and boost sales" (Meskin, 1997, p. 264). It was the dentists, Meskin contended "not the public who are the victims" (p. 265). He continued to say that the variance that Ecenbarger identified might have reflected dentists' frames of reference to oral disease and their treatment preferences. Finally, he concluded that the public should be aware of cost differences in aesthetic vs. restorative dentistry.

Roger Levin (1997), CEO of a dental management and marketing firm, responded with an article in *Dental Economics*. In a sidebar he offered practitioners five "quick and dirty strategies for countering negative press" (p. 32). He expressed concern that Ecenbarger (1997) did not consider issues that could potentially influence the range and cost of a dentist's treatment plan such as scope and quality of services rendered, geographical location, amenities provided, expertise and experience of the dentist, and technology used in diagnosis and treatment. The president of the American Dental Association, Gary

Rainwater, called the article a "character assassination of an entire profession" (Kehoe & Blunk, 1997, p. 24). In the same article, another clinician questioned the ethics of Ecenbarger in not telling the dentists the true nature of his visit. Following this was a call to address the important ethical issue that Ecenbarger raised. On the other hand, W. W. Oakes, editor of *The Profitable Dentist Newsletter,* questioned whether Ecenbarger understood the nature of the exams he underwent. He disagreed with the journalist that the dentists visited were more interested in their profits than the patient's dental health. Finally, sampling in this article was questioned: "I have to believe that the author hand-picked dentists who were known to be dishonest or incompetent" (Kehoe & Blunk, 1997, p. 28).

It will be years before the full impact of this article on dentistry is revealed. How the profession responds is critical. Many initial reactions have been defensive in nature, while others propose methods of "damage control". Members of the profession must work together and seek some form of consensus to account for what is happening, and then truly identify the problem. This is more than just a "public relations fiasco". It is suggested that dental leaders chart a course of corporate responsibility (not spin) to regain their consumers' trust.

IS DEPENDABILITY AN OPTION?

There is no alternative to being dependable, reliable, and responsible in establishing trust in our personal and professional relationships. Daily headlines feature individuals who try to evade the responsibility of their actions. For the pain, cost, and/or irritation they cause, there is always someone else to blame. Witness a 1997 public radio feature regarding a disbarred New England attorney and his pursuit to retain his right to practice.

The lawyer in question had his license suspended for 3 years. There was considerable evidence against him concerning dependability and responsibility, and this cost others considerable time, money, and effort. He was late submitting or never filed his paperwork. Tardiness and absenteeism with court appearances, client meetings, and even picking up his kids from school were the routine. In some cases he loaned money of one client to another without the first client's knowledge. Judges, court officials, clients, and many others were furious. Trials and hearings were delayed or postponed, and people lost their cases because of missed deadlines.

Unfortunately, this was not the end. This attorney held degrees from Ivy League colleges, earned a Rhodes

Scholarship, and had been elected to the state assembly. To regain his law license, he appealed his case to the state's Supreme Court because of new evidence on his behalf. These events were not his fault, he claimed, as he was just diagnosed with attention deficit disorder. Under the Americans with Disabilities Act, his new "disability" will serve as both his defense and excuse for years of irresponsible practice behavior.

There must be a greater commitment to personal responsibility. Citizens must have confidence in providers and be able to count on them to do what they are supposed to do and be where they are supposed to be. Can we no longer believe what others say? Does personal responsibility extend only as far as what can be gotten away with? Dependability is not an option. It only becomes an option if we decide to let trust fall from our vocabulary.

Background

Some of the basic ingredients for a dependable health career include a sound professional education, effective planning skills, and expertise in time management. Over the years I have attended numerous community and professional award ceremonies. While some received highest honors for cutting edge performance or working beyond the call of duty, most were recognized for their day to day attention to detail in approaching their responsibilities. In other words, the latter group was awarded for being dependable. Several of the acceptance speeches I witnessed opened with the following comment: "I don't know why I am being recognized for this award. I didn't do anything special; I was only doing my job." As we will see, their grasp of dependability is what has made them better communicators, organizers, and/or supervisors. In the end, they gained the trust of those they served.

Related Literature

PROFESSIONAL EDUCATION AND MORE

What is a health care professional? Addressing counselors, Spurill and Benshoff (1996) present a composite definition of professionalism, including "internalized attitudes, perspectives, and personal commitment to the standards, ideals, and identity of a profession". They go on to cite evidence of professionalism, including "active participation and leadership in professional organizations, acquisition of appropriate counselor credentials, professional growth, and continued pursuit of knowledge" (p. 468).

The basic thrust of professional education is to impart the intellectual and psychomotor skills necessary to practice. The path of learning includes both prerequisite and professional coursework, accompanied by a clinical component that varies according to field. Out of practical necessity, students, faculty, and clinical supervisors often focus on the performance and cognitive components of education. The more intangible constructs of empathy and initiative, for example, may receive less attention. It may inaccurately be assumed that they will pick up these qualities through casual observation. Therefore it is possible to have a provider with substantial cognitive knowledge but limitations in cooperation and dependability. It may take awhile for these deficits to become obvious in one's professional career.

It should be clear that success in building consumer confidence is not due to professional knowledge and skill alone. From the patient's perspective a provider's diagnostic and treatment skills are a given, the result of going to medical, nursing, or therapy school, for instance. What is important to these patients is the way they are treated as people. It is the relationship with their provider and the provider's character that counts. Recall the results of the patient survey from earlier in the chapter. Beyond professional skills, they want a provider who can be counted upon under all conditions. If patients don't see this, they will take their business elsewhere.

Issues where character augments skill are also critical in education. Meier (1994) lists the three Rs where she stresses resilience, reliability, and sense of responsibility. She is founder and director of an East Harlem alternative public high school in New York City. Her students graduate and go on to college at a substantially higher rate than the rest of the city's students as a whole. Resilience, reliability, and sense of responsibility are the habits of the mind and character that will determine her students' futures far more than SAT scores and grade point average.

PROFESSIONAL PLANNING AND OUR "LIFE PURPOSE"

Professionals must develop dependable life and work styles. This will have to occur under mandates of health care reform where efficiency and profit require us to do more with less. Now more than ever we must be able to count on our fellow professionals for consistency in teamwork. There may be few checks and balances with what one does, and final accountability may be to the agencies paying the bills.

Jones' (1996) work is particularly directed to developing dependability. According to her thesis, we must discern important activities from the less important. It is our mission statement that defines our life purpose, and it remains relatively constant. Through this we set our priorities. Once in place, the mission statement serves as a filter through which we screen every choice, activity, and opportunity. With continuous filtering we get ever closer to attaining our life purpose. This is because we do only that which contributes to the accomplishment of our purpose. Over time our priority setting and decision-making become efficient and effective.

THE MISSION STATEMENT

Determining one's mission statement is beyond the scope of this chapter. Briefly, these statements vary from person to person. Individuals in the same field might develop dramatically different mission statements. It does not come overnight. We base it on our past experience, our projected resources, our inner desires, and our dreams. A nurse, for example, might want to prolong life in the emphysemic elderly, find a solution to poverty related childhood diseases, or promote the health care of women and children. Conversely she may have chosen nursing as a means to increase social and financial security for her family. She may wish to be able to travel and photograph marshlands wildlife or write the great American novel. With a mission statement in place, our short-term goals and priorities will evolve and become refined as we pursue our life purpose.

If our life purpose is not clear and we attempt too many paths, our professional life will become chaotic. We chance making too many altruistic decisions for the wrong reasons or too many obligatory commitments that leave us frazzled but do not further our mission. We become stretched too thin, and we are seen as unreliable or irresponsible. Or we may spin our wheels endlessly dealing just with the tyranny of the urgent.

ONE CONCEPT OF TIME MANAGEMENT: MARGIN

Predictions were made years ago that by the end of the 20th Century, Americans would be working less and enjoying it more. We all know this has not happened. In fact, the opposite is occurring, and our battle with time is

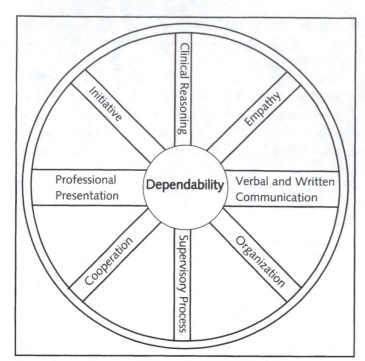

Figure 4-1. Dependability, the hub of professional behaviors.

just being declared. Beepers, timers, cell phones, e-mail, and alarms give us nothing but stress. Time should not be our enemy, dictating our every move, cramping our style, and causing us to rush around. Quality time in personal and family life will make our professional time with patients more effective. Physician Richard Swenson (1992) proposes the concept of margin with respect to time. Margin is the extra space between us and our limits, a buffer zone. It gives us energy, calm, and security. Rarely can one accurately predict the end of a workday, and this plays havoc on family life. Thus, my wife calls me between 4:30-5:00 PM for my estimate. I usually add 20 extra minutes of margin to when I think I will be home, and I am glad that I do this. Things I have put off or unexpected events have a way of creeping into my schedule that would otherwise make me late every night.

To restore our time margin, Swenson (1992) offers the following: always allow more time than is expected in your planning. If one chain in the event is delayed, you will be glad you did. If you are habitually late, and you know who you are, build an extra 20 minutes into the schedule. Learn to say no. You cannot do everything you are asked to do. Practice simplicity in your possessions and lifestyle. Complex "things" and "toys" require time, energy, and money to maintain. Formulate a long-term plan. Going hour by hour or day by day is chaotic and hectic at best.

According to Swenson, we must change the mindset that we should do more in less time. Instead, he suggests, it is better to get less done, but to do the right things. Do not rush decisions—important ones take time. Get time away from the workplace to eat, browse, or enjoy solitude and leisure. For health care professionals, he recommends inserting an "imaginary patient" into the schedule. This is a definite no-show, which will allow a free time slot to catch up and/or recoup (1992). This allows the time needed for documentation, for new policies, upcoming reaccreditation visits, or other report requirements. How many of us know professionals, both inside and outside of health care, who earn considerable incomes but have no time to spend and enjoy what they make? The fascinating concepts of time theory, work, and leisure are beyond the scope here, but a classic reference on time is by de Grazia (1962).

DEPENDABILITY AS THE HUB OF PROFESSIONAL BEHAVIOR

The meaning of dependability has been presented. It remains intricately intertwined with personal responsibility, reliability, and most importantly, it is the foundation for trust. It is understood that dependability is a necessary quality for success in practice. But what is its relationship to other professional behaviors? Dependability is important in all we do, but why? Consider the analogy of the wheel in Figure 4-1. The wheel is free to spin on its axle. The outer rim represents a successful practice. Each spoke is a basic professional behavior (as labeled). Spokes provide the strength, balance, and stability of the wheel. With a missing spoke or two, the other spokes will take the load, and the wheel will continue to function. However, it will be less efficient. Dependability is at the center of the wheel—it is the hub. It connects the other professional behaviors to one another and serves as the base of support for every spoke. With a broken hub, the spokes will slowly fall out of place and reduce the integrity of the wheel until it collapses. It is the hub of dependability in which each of the professional behaviors has its grounding. Remove the hub and there can be no successful professional practice.

How Dependability is Developed

Problems in Dependability Do Matter— Recognize Them

The majority of health care professionals have little difficulty with dependability issues. However, when there is a problem, and it can be career threatening, immediate recognition is necessary. "Responsibility is a difficult thing to talk about. It is often seen as something that others should have more of; few of us think of ourselves as irresponsible" (Souba, 1996, p. 7). Awareness of the problem usually reaches us in some form of feedback from our supervisor or in a complaint from a patient. Sometimes this brings in defensiveness and this can make matters worse. Because dependability is the hub that holds the other professional behaviors in place, its deficit can negatively influence growth in other areas, such as communication, organization, or supervision.

DEPENDABILITY AT HOME

Dependability in professional life is extremely important, but it can be just as critical in matters at home. Consider the consequences of not addressing the following: timely payment of the rent, mortgage, taxes, and utilities; maintenance of the car with yearly state safety inspections; picking up the kids from day care; ensuring children's immunizations and school registrations; repairing leaks when first noticed; keeping up on lawn care or shoveling the snow from the sidewalk; making regular insurance installments; paying the paperboy. Dependability is a rather universal construct with pragmatic implications. In the old Chinese proverb it is stated: "Dependable at home, dependable at work". Unfortunately, the converse is also true.

A SELF-ASSESSMENT

At the end of this chapter is a self-assessment for dependability based on issues associated with dependability. It is not the intent of this instrument to reveal a score for comparison to norms or peers. Instead, the items are meant to provoke thought and introspection. It is best to address this assessment while alone. Write out your answers. After some thought, share your findings with a mentor or peer. It is a time for honesty. Your "why's" and "why not's" for each item are more important than your "yes" or "no". Look for trends in your answers.

THE PROCESS OF CHANGE

Identification and acknowledgement of problems in dependability become the foundation for change. Feedback from a supervisor, peer, or even your results on the self-assessment may convey that there is an issue. Bill was a speech pathologist who noticed that the secretary was becoming rather gruff with him. This went on over time until he discussed it at lunch with a colleague. The colleague suggested that he approach the secretary and find out what was going on. When he did, she blew up at him, as she was angry at his tardiness in submitting all his reports and waiting until the end of the month. This was when everything else was due for her. And she was tired of defending him from repeated agency calls questioning the delay of her reports. While the secretary had a problem in communication, Bill was not dependable in timely report preparation. He subsequently admitted to his procrastination and appropriately revised his working habits.

Upon acknowledgement must come the motivation and energy to do something positive to change. Detailed theories about motivation and transition to change are well documented in counseling and psychological literature. For the purpose of this text, I make the following recommendation: set a personal goal to be viewed as trustworthy, and you will become dependable. Obtaining one's trust is a strong motivator toward developing many professional behaviors. As a broad jumper on the track team, I was told that the way to increase my distance was to aim for height as I jumped. If you want to be dependable, aim for trust. This is an excellent source of motivation. This follows an old proverb that is most appropriate here: "The only thing better than a trusted friend is a friend who trusts you".

Role Modeling/Mentorship

The best mentoring for dependability is to model the appropriate behaviors during a student's clinical experience. As seasoned practitioners, we sometimes go out of our way to insure that our health care plan is carried out. If we take these steps when a student tags alongside, it is important that we point these out to them as examples of dependable behaviors.

Consider the following. Take the time to call for the Spanish translator even though the patient nods and smiles in understanding when receiving instructions. Show Mrs. Smith her new exercises for yet another time when her daughter comes in to pick her up, knowing that the daughter will accurately follow the instructions. Provide Mr. Jones with three alternatives of the same thing, knowing that he will be more compliant if he makes the choice. Schedule an elderly lady right before lunch because if more time is needed, her treatment won't run into another's session. Call a new patient at the end of the day with some reassurance. Refuse to take an additional patient when this will impact on the quality of care given to others. Emphasize attention to detail and diligence when charting or preparing other reports. If students repeatedly observe these acts and how they positively impact your practice, they will add them to their repertoire. Be sure that you follow through with your offers and promises made to the student, as well as being timely and punctual in all your interactions.

Patient Dependability

BASIC ISSUES

Discussions in this chapter have addressed personal, home, and corporate dependability. But to ensure a patients' compliance to a wellness or treatment plan, they too must be dependable, as they follow instructions and report changes in their symptomatology. With increased trust in the provider, patients become more open in communication, more diligent in carrying out doctor's, nurse's, or therapist's orders. A phenomenon that reduces the effectiveness of treatment is when patients say what they think the practitioner wants to hear as they report back. We rely on their feedback in order to adjust their treatment plan if the current scheme is not working. "Paul, I did not want you to feel bad, you worked so hard on my wrist... but it is still sore; I just couldn't tell you." In another situation a patient may report success rather than face an alternate treatment or procedure that is not of their choosing. Finally, there are compliance issues. "I'm so sorry, but I could not get those pills down. I was afraid that you would be angry at me." Whether it is medication, exercise, rest, or another care plan, mutual trust and dependability between patient and provider are the best means to promote compliance.

It is also important to solicit a patients' opinion when there are choices to be made. If, in your opinion, a patients' contribution to the care plan is not an appropriate one, probe further before you respond. Consider their perspective. What are their goals? What are their social, employment, financial, and time variables? Do they have time constraints? There may be some data missing in your clinical reasoning equation, which, if known to you, could make the patients' suggestions more feasible. The more we learn about our patients, the more flexible our frames of reference become.

Reconsider the patients' perspective. Try to determine where they are coming from. Some may want an author-

ity figure to lead while they follow along, e.g., "Tell me what to do, and I will do it." Another patient may want most of the responsibility herself with peripheral guidance from the provider. "Can't I carry out my therapy at home, and keep you posted by phone?" Then there are patients who want a quick repair, just sufficient to function at home and work, and they will carry out the remainder of the plan from there. "Please do not do any more than you have to in order to get me back to work." Others may want full, but mutual, involvement until maximum medical improvement has been achieved.

With rising costs and shrinking benefits, some patients may not be able to afford the plan as presented, but are too proud to admit this to you and so they go away. Culture, language, family issues, pain tolerance, age, gender, and secondary gain, for example, may each impact a patient's contribution and subsequent compliance in the care plan. Talk to the patients about their ideas and concerns. Sometimes it requires no more than a clarification of a procedure to obtain the optimum patient/provider match. Facilitate their personal responsibility. Sharpen their observation skills. Ask, "Do you have a sense of what your body is telling you and can you try to explain it to me?" In using this approach, it is important not to put words into their mouths. Instead, help them express the right terms.

Some clinicians are skeptical about using self-report data because of reliability considerations, and there is some basis for this reservation. Open communication between provider and patient remains an efficient means to foster efficacy, trust, and patient responsibility throughout the evaluation and treatment process.

A PATIENT/CONSUMER

An excellent example of a patient/consumer is Connie, a middle-aged woman who sustained a fall away from home. This resulted primarily in long-term and almost fatal central nervous system, articular, and sensory disorders. She underwent surgery and extensive rehabilitation, both as an inpatient and outpatient. Fortunately, her communication and cognitive capacities were largely spared, and graduate degrees in medical sociology contributed to her sophistication throughout the ordeal. Once stabilized and home, she sought new specialists for follow-up. Given the complexity of her problems, she interacted with a number of medical specialists and requested to interview each before accepting them as part of her team. She was not as interested in their credentials as she was in having trusting relationships with two-way communication. She was always willing to help with literature research.

Given the above scenario, one might assume Connie to be an excessively demanding, critical, and complaining individual. But in actuality, she was none of these. She made contributions that were incorporated into her therapy, and they were right on target. She was receptive to suggestions. Overall, she was highly compliant, motivated, and open. Simply put, she wanted a part of the responsibility for her own rehabilitation plan, and she took it.

LOWERING THE WALL

As health care professionals, we assume some degree of autonomy and authority in our patient/provider interaction. This can be viewed as a wall or gap that separates us from those we serve. As patients take on some of the responsibility for their care, the locus of control shifts proportionately away from the provider. Some professionals fear this change in balance will threaten their autonomy and reduce their authority, serving to undermine their effectiveness. They lack comfort when lowering the wall or narrowing this patient/provider gap.

I am not stating that we tear down the wall or fill in the gap completely. What I do offer is that we can lower the wall or narrow the gap and still maintain our comfort from the trust derived by the shared responsibility for the patient's care. We may not always understand the weight of the burden we have in the patient's eyes. They see us for important and personal reasons, and their expectations of our capabilities may be more than what is humanly possible. No matter what we do, our best may not be enough for them, and we will fail in their eyes. We should clarify patient expectations from the start and then realistically correlate them with our own capabilities and intentions. This is responsible practice.

Malpractice and Dependability

THE COST

As already stated, there is a cost when dependability is lacking. Deficits here prevent the forming of trustful interpersonal relationships with patients. For many providers, it is the richness of these relationships that is the most important part of their work. Lacking this satisfaction is most regrettable. However, there are more tangible outcomes beyond limited job dissatisfaction. They range from loss of income or job to a lawsuit. Medical malpractice is an industry. There is much to be learned from the literature, as deficiencies in dependability, trust, and other topics in this book are the root causes for many lawsuits.

In the ever-growing research on litigation, there are several reasons that cause the physicians and nurses to be most often sued. They are usually the closest to life and death issues, they carry greater liability insurance, and they are often the focus of the patient's anger and frustration. Others in the health care field are not immune from litigation. Barium swallow and video fluoroscopic studies, for example, offer potential risk for speech pathologists. As such, most allied health providers today carry malpractice insurance. It is important to understand that it is both harm-causing behaviors and follow-up attitudes that usually bring us to court. Familiarization with these behaviors and attitudes will make us better practitioners.

SOME ARE SUED AND OTHERS ARE NOT

In general, poor outcomes prompt patients to sue their providers. There is, however, a paradox. Not all adverse outcomes result in suits, and not all lawsuits involve maloccurrence (Beckman, Markakis, Suchman, & Frankel, 1994). The study by Beckman, et. al. found support for this paradox in relationship issues between practitioner and patient. Following some undue suffering, many patients and/or families felt deserted and alone. Practitioners rarely responded to their needs or calls. Others did not keep promises to return to the bedside. Few solicited patient or family opinion, and many were inattentive to the patient's discomfort. Many delivered information poorly, skipping over the "what's and why's" of a procedure. In all these examples, a breakdown in trust accompanied the alleged medical maloccurrence. Given this atmosphere, combined with untoward results, anger and suspicion are raised. Patients and families start to murmur, "What are they trying to hide, and what are they trying to get away with?" Many examples of this paradox are found in Leaman & Saxton (1993).

WHY DO PATIENTS SUE?

Vincent, Young, and Phillips (1994) surveyed 227 patients and surviving family members in the United Kingdom and extrapolated four factors why legal action was taken. In the first factor, *accountability*, there is the consideration that a practitioner or institution should be held responsible. *Compensation* as a factor represents a sum of money offered for financial loss or suffering, etc. *Explanation* is based on feeling ignored or neglected after the incident. They want to know what happened and why. *Standards of care* conveys the patient's or family's desire to prevent a similar incident from happening to another individual.

Forty-one percent of the litigants in the same study identified actions after the maloccurrence that might have prevented them from suing. Several of their reasons were an explanation or apology, correction of the mistake, admission of negligence, honesty, openness to listen to the complaint, and not being treated as a neurotic. Deficiencies in communication are manifested in unsympathetic and unclear explanations. Appreciating the emotional needs of one's patients may be just as important as treating their physical needs (Vincent, et al., 1994). Poor interpersonal relationships remain a key factor in malpractice. Huycke & Huycke (1994) characterized a large sample of patients phoning plaintiff attorneys' offices claiming to have suffered injuries caused by medical negligence. The researchers anticipated that potential plaintiffs would be angry with their providers after the untoward incident. This was true. Most felt that they were not being kept informed or appropriately referred. Surprisingly, however, they found that 53% identified unsatisfactory relationships before the alleged injury!

These findings emphasize over and over again that patients demand more than our professional knowledge; they already assume we have this. They want providers who care about them, express an interest in them, and go out of their way to advance their health status. Deficiencies in these responsibilities account for some lawsuits in the absence of a maloccurrence. Our attitudes and behaviors must change for the better. We have to work closer with our patients and insure meaningful communication and attitudes of care.

THE CO-ACTIVE SOLUTION

Thomas Leaman, a physician, described two cases of malpractice from his own caseload for which he was not sued. He was always open with his patients and tried to incorporate their views and support them whenever possible. He stated that on the face of his two actions, were he the judge or juror in either case, and based on these actions alone, he would have ruled against himself and on the side of the patient in each (Leaman & Saxton, 1993).

Leaman offers advice to others in his book, co-authored with attorney James Saxton, on preventing malpractice (Leaman & Saxton, 1993). They suggest an alternative to defensive health care and risk management and call theirs the co-active solution. Simply stated, the doctor and patient work together to improve the patient's health. The physician tells the patient that they will collaborate as a partnership and they each have their responsibilities. Differing from risk management, here the patient becomes a partner instead of an adversary. "Co-active practice provides the format, the structure, for the kind of personalized care that people crave. It also provides the doctor with a consultant who can give information that cannot be found anywhere else — what does the patient want to do?"(p. 92).

Not all patients will immediately adapt to this co-active approach. Some will want the provider to assume all the responsibility and risk. Another might state "You're in charge, why are you asking me what we should do?" Should you invite patient cooperation and responsibility, be sure you sincerely consider what they tell you. While sitting in a waiting room, I overheard a patient comment to his wife as they left the office, "Why did she bother asking me what I thought when she really doesn't care?" If your solicitations are seen as shallow and insincere, you are certain to lose their trust.

Case Stories/Anecdotal Vignettes

As you read through the following cases and narratives, identify examples of dependability or its absence. How does each case illustrate the definitions given in the chapter? Which, if any, of the vignettes relate to the professional's psychomotor skills vs. his or her attitudes and trustworthiness? What is learned from the positive scenarios? How might this vignette apply to your clinical situation? For the negatives, what could have been done to insure a better outcome? How was patient care impacted? What influenced the building of patient/provider interaction and most ultimately, trust, or lack of, in that relationship?

Lack of Dependability and Its Effects

OH, MY ACHING SHOULDER

John, a 73-year-old man in good health, came in for therapy following complex surgery to reconstruct his shoulder.

The local doctor told me my rotator cuff was really in bad shape after years of abuse, but he was able to repair it. I was to go easy on my rehab. He sent me for therapy, and that was the start of my problems. All my therapy consisted of was exercise, and I was usually on my own, just me, my clipboard, and the machine, that bloody machine. There was little attempt to address the pain. I never liked my therapy assistant. She was cocky, and I did not feel like she was that experienced. Anyway, she was having a quarrel over the phone with her boyfriend one day during my therapy. I had a question about one of the new exercises and wanted her to show me the correct procedure. She just waved me off and told me to do it. It was easy, she said. I attempted it, and I may have done it wrong. My shoulder made a loud popping sound. The pain was severe and unrelenting. This went on for over a month until they figured out what was going on. I could not move the arm at all. So I had to see a specialist out of state to reconstruct the thing.

TOO MANY CHAIRS

A colleague complained about his dentist of several years having too many chairs in the office. *He jumps from examining room to room making us wait long periods in between his short visits. There is no need to pack us in like that. During one appointment he returned from a break stating "How's Bill? Now let's finish filling that cavity." My name isn't Bill, and I was having a crown put on. He is either too busy or trying to make too much money, I don't know which. I guess his dental work is all right, and he is very friendly. But I am afraid he may do the wrong procedure one day or forget to change his gloves. I finally got another dentist.*

HAVING THE HEART FOR LUNCH

A middle-aged woman related her experience in dealing with her father's cardiac surgeon. *My dad was getting very tired. Thinking it was his age (73) he ignored it at first. He needed further medical testing, which identified a silent heart attack and other conditions requiring bypass surgery. After one series of tests, the doctor, dressed in scrubs and lab coat, told us the results were in, and he would be right back to review the findings and his plans before we went home. We had been there almost 5 hours already. My father had neither food nor water since awakening early that morning. Because of this he had not yet taken his heart mediation, and he's a diabetic. We were all very nervous. More than an hour and a half later the surgeon reappeared, this time in a busi-*

ness suit. Apparently he went out for lunch. I do not know what came over me, but I read him the riot act about my father being kept waiting so long while he took off. Then I wished I had not said the things I did, as he would be the surgeon doing the bypass. Everything got quiet. He neither commented nor apologized. As we left the hospital, the nurse quietly commented to me, "I am glad you said that to the doctor; he does that a lot. We can't say anything, but he needs to hear about it."

Presence of Dependability and Effects

DUELING HOSPITALS

A man in his late sixties related the following narrative. *I wouldn't recommend a dog to Central Hospital. The nursing care there was terrible the last time my wife was in. They never answered her call bell when she needed her pain pills. When she rang a second time an hour later, an angry nurse appeared with an attitude, like the pain was in my wife's head or something. The whole experience was a nightmare. Fortunately, she came out alright. For my last operation my doctor offered me the choice of either hospital. I chose University Hospital this time. The operation was risky but successful. The nurses were wonderful. They went out of their way to be helpful. I can't say enough about that place. I hope never to go again, but if I have to, it's University for me. I've told all my friends.*

CONCERN FOR HIS PATIENT'S TIME

A referring surgeon has an international reputation and was busily engaged in professional activity, necessitating limited office hours with long waits. But his patients do not complain, but rather only praise him. A synopsis of the comments heard over the years follow, "In addition to being the best surgeon, I never feel rushed when it is my turn, he answers my questions, and he has a great sense of humor." One specific comment worth mentioning was that the doctor is "like a good restaurant. He's worth the drive and the wait. He really knows what my elbow is all about." This doctor values the patient's time as much as his own. As many travel long distances, the surgeon encourages them to call ahead to his office to see if there is a delay and how long it will be, so that they can adjust their time of departure from home. This cuts their waiting time down significantly. For a while his staff allowed long distance patients to register for their appointment by phone, further reducing their wait. Unfortunately, this policy was abused and subsequently rescinded by the office staff.

THAT EXTRA STEP

A middle-aged woman had a long-standing oral motor problem that presented no long-term health threat. There is not a lot known about her condition, and it is approached symptomatically. She was seeing a local ear, nose, and throat physician for treatment as needed and had great confidence in him. One day at work her excitement was showing. She recently received a call from her doctor at home. He had just returned from a medical conference and very new information on the course and treatment of her condition was addressed. She immediately came to his mind, and he was sending her three articles resulting from a computer search. If she was willing to consider some of the new procedures, he was ready to try and/or refer her to some nationally known specialists.

References

Beckman, H. B., Markakis, K. M., Suchman, A. L., & Frankel, R. M. (1994). The doctor-patient relationship and malpractice: Lessons from plaintiff depositions. *Archives of Internal Medicine, 54*, 1365-1370.

Coy, L. (1985). *Quotable quotations*. Wheaton, Il: Victor.

Crook, P. L. (1994). Worker's compensation. In C. D. Tollison (Ed.), *Handbook of pain management*, Second ed. (pp. 722-731). Baltimore, MD: Williams & Wilkins.

de Grazia, S. (1962). *Of time, work, and leisure*. New York, NY: Twentieth Century Fund.

Ecenbarger, W. (1997). How honest are dentists? *Reader's Digest, 150* (898, February), 50-56.

Flaherty, J. A. (1985). Attitudinal development in medical education. In A. Rezler & J. A. Flaherty (Eds.), *The interpersonal dimension in medical education* (pp.147-182). New York, NY: Springer.

Husted, B. W. (1993). Reliability and the design of ethical organizations: A rational systems approach. *Journal of Business Ethics, 12*, 761-769.

Huycke, L. I., & Huycke, M. M. (1994). Characteristics of potential plaintiffs in malpractice litigation. *Annals of Internal Medicine, 129*, 792-798.

Jones, L. B. (1996). *The path*. New York, NY: Hyperion.

Kececiogly, D. (1991). *Reliability engineering handbook: Vol 1.* Englewood Cliffs, NJ: Prentice Hall.

Kehoe, B., & Blunk, D. (1997). Target practice: Why Reader's Digest threw darts at dentistry. *Dental Practice & Finance*, (March/April), 24-25, 28.

Leaman, T. L., & Saxton, J. W. (1993). *Preventing malpractice: The co-active solution*. New York, NY: Plenum.

Levin, R. (1997). Your reply to Reader's Digest. *Dental Economics*, (March), 30, 32, 34.

Meier, D. (1994). A talk to teachers on resilience, reliability, and a sense of responsibility. *Dissent* (Winter), 80-87.

Meskin, L. H. (1997). Editorial: A dental rip-off. *Journal of the American Dental Association, 238*, 264-266.

Moorman, C., Deshpande, R., & Zaltman, G. (1993). Factors affecting trust in market research relationships. *Journal of Marketing, 57*, 81-101.

Souba, W. W. (1996). Professionalism, responsibility, and service in academic medicine. *Surgery, 119*, 1-8.

Spurill, D. A., & Benshoff J. M. (1996). The future is now: Promoting professionalism among counselors-in-training. *Journal of Counseling & Development, 74*, 468-471.

Swenson, R. A. (1992). *Margin: How to create the emotional, physical, financial, and time reserves you need*. Colorado Springs, CO: Navpress.

Vincent, C., Young, M., & Phillips, A. (1994). Why do people sue doctors? A study of patients and relatives taking legal action. *Lancet, 343*, 1609-1613.

Exercises to Develop Dependability

Exercise 1: Self-Assessment on Dependability for Health Care Professionals

Directions: Take sufficient time to complete the following assessment. Purposefully consider the "why's" and "why not's" of your answers, and explore appropriate feedback from others whenever possible.

1.) Did I meet all my appointments today relatively on time? Was my schedule realistic?

2.) Did I give any excuses to anyone today? If so, were my excuses valid?

3.) Is all my paperwork and administration accurate and up-to-date at the end of the workday?

4.) When I go to a clinic for personal and family needs and endure a long wait, how do I react?

5.) Did I see to it that all appropriate phone, fax, or email messages from staff and patients asking for responses were taken care of today?

6.) Do I really understand the theoretical basis and practical application of the procedures I performed today?

7.) Are my theoretical understanding and my fine motor skills sufficient to do what is required?

8.) Was there any need or reason for me to request a second opinion or consult a colleague today? Did I do so? If not, why?

9.) Did a patient ask for more time than I could give today? Was his or her expressed need realistic? What did I do about the request?

10.) Do I ever work when I am sick? If so, do I put my patients at risk?

11.) Do I feel overworked? Do I find I'm excessively tired during or by the end of my workday?

12.) Did I treat each patient today as I, or members of my family, would like to be treated?

13.) Did I make a mistake or cause pain or harm today? Did I apologize and try to make things right?

14.) Did I make promises to others? Did I keep my promises to patients, colleagues, or staff members?

15.) Was there someone today for whom I could have done more, but did not? Why not?

16.) Could I honestly tell each patient that I've done my best for him or her?

17.) Was I satisfied with my work today?

Exercise 2.

Arrange with a clinical supervisor to conduct short interviews with a few patients at your setting. Ask them to name are some of the most important characteristics they look for when they seek a health care professional. Which of their answers have to do with trust, dependability, and self-responsibility? Is it important to hear this from a patient? Was there anything you heard that will change the way you conduct your professional career?

Exercise 3.

Peruse your local newspaper for feature stories, community interest, editorials, and letters to the editor. In which can you identify where dependability and responsibility stand out, where is it lacking? Where dependability is lacking, what are your recommendations for change or for prevention? In the positive stories, what can be done to perpetuate dependability? Our Saturday newspaper issues a weekly acknowledgement to a local citizen who has dependably served a cause. Look in your hometown paper for such recognition.

Exercise 4.

In a group setting, ask fellow students to cite examples from their clinic on the topic of dependability; include both positive and negative. Discuss each. How did the observing students respond? Were they in a position to contribute to the issue? How was the issue resolved, or was it resolved? What did the students learn from this experience?

Exercise 5.

Returning to the newspaper, identify a story involving dependability (either pro or con), and draft a Letter to the Editor in response to the story. Review the printed letters as examples, and check the small print for proper format. Why did you identify this story? What will be the main theme(s) of your response? Consider submitting it.

Additional Resources

Byerly, L. D. (1996). How do patients define "service." *Health Progress* (July-August). 95-96.

Cloud, H., & Townsend, J. (1992). *Boundaries: When to say YES, when to say NO to take control of your life.* Grand Rapids, MI: Zondervan. (Author's note: There is a workbook that accompanies this text.)

Purtilo, R. B., & Cassel, C. K. (1981). *Ethical dimensions in the health professions.* Philadelphia, PA: Saunders.

Saxton, J. W. (1995). *Satisfied patient: A guide to preventing claims and promoting managed care goals.* Lancaster, PA: Worldwide Media.

Wallace, R. J. (1994). *Responsibility and the moral sentiments.* Cambridge, MA: Harvard.

Zimmerman, M. J. (1996). *Concepts of moral obligation.* New York, NY: Cambridge.

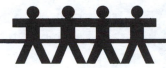

Chapter Five

Professional Presentation

Jan Larkey

Seven Seconds to Image Impact

Being successful in your chosen health care field depends on more than credentials. Whether you are just beginning your career or seeking advancement, it pays to understand the major impact your image has on getting a job, promotions, raises—and most importantly—your effectiveness with your patients.

What is an image? An image is the total impression created by a person. It includes your appearance, posture, body language, speech patterns, voice, and even your attitude. Research shows when prospective employers or patients first see you, you have only 7 seconds to make a first impression (Fleschner, 1995). Thereafter, you will be evaluated against that initial reaction. Interviewers decide in the first few minutes if you will be hired or passed over; the rest of the interview is spent justifying that first impression. It is extremely difficult to reverse a bad first impression.

Your boss, colleagues, and patients respond to you as a result of assumptions and attitudes they form about you based on your physical appearance. Behavioral scientists have conducted hundreds of studies verifying that physical appearance variables such as physical attractiveness, weight, height, facial characteristics, and grooming factors affect attitudes and actions (Cash, 1990).

To test the "7 second" theory, glance at the woman in Figure 5-1, and then answer the questions below.

1. How old is she?

2. How much education has she completed?

3. What type of job does she have?

4. What is her annual salary?

5. Will she get a raise or promotion this year?

6. How does she feel about herself?

Your answers probably reflect those of numerous audiences who have seen this picture. They typically think she is between 40 and 50. She has, at most, a high school diploma or the GED. She works in a cafeteria line, as a grocery store cashier, or on an assembly line, making minimum wage or about $12,000 a year. She will not be promoted, and she appears to have very low self-esteem.

Now glance at Figure 5-2 and answer the same questions as above.

The real answers to the first picture are:

1. 40
2. Master's degree from Stanford University
3. Unsuccessful job hunting: Art Teacher
4. Previous salary: $15,000 (1980)
5. Standard raise—if teaching!
6. Low self-esteem

Most audiences are shocked to discover that these two pictures are the same woman, except in the second picture I am 10 years older. Yes, this is my picture. What made the difference? After failing to get a job in 1980, I changed my appearance and it changed my professional life. Instead of looking pitiful, I packaged myself on the outside to reflect the real me—a competent woman with the education and abilities to do a good job.

Figure 5-1. Seven second theory example 1.

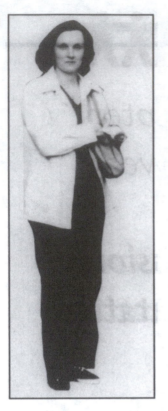

Figure 5-2. Seven second theory example 2.

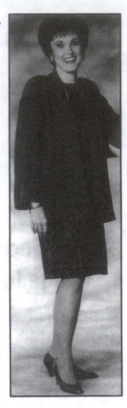

According to communication expert Roger Ailes, who has counseled Fortune 500 professionals and is the CEO of CNBC, our instant evaluations of people we meet are a primitive reaction to signals sent by that person (Fleschner, 1980, p. 14). In caveman days, you had only seconds to react to whether a stranger was friend or foe. Reading the signals wrong could cost you your life. Today, sending the wrong signals can cost you a job or the confidence of your patients.

What signals are you sending? Do you look friendly? Competent? Trustworthy? Caring? Confident? Or is your visual message keeping you from meeting your goals, just as mine once did?

The matter of creating a positive image is not a shallow, vain, or phony effort to please a boss or make someone think you are something you are not. It is a vital part of being a professional. Your appearance is a business tool that can open or close doors of opportunity for you. It shows others how you value yourself—and them. The message your visual impact sends is the first connection between the patient and you, the caregiver. It sets the tone for all future communication.

While you may not like it, your first impression counts more than how competently you perform your job, states William Thourlby (1978) in his book *You Are What You*

Wear; even more than all the time and effort you spent to become well-educated in your chosen profession.

Would you go back to see a dentist who had diplomas hanging all over his walls but wore a dirty lab coat and had halitosis? Of course not. The impression people form when they first see you will determine if your patients respect you as a professional.

The key to creating a positive first impression is to understand what your body language and appearance instantly communicate to others about you.

Body Language

Messages about yourself are sent both verbally and non-verbally. What you say to a patient can be reinforced—or negated—by non-verbal visual clues from your body language. According to Albert Mehrabian (1981) in his book *Silent Messages*, when your body language is not consistent with what you are saying, the message people believe will be based 55% on your facial expression (visual impact), 38% on the tone of your voice (vocal impact), and only 7% on the actual words you say (verbal impact).

Consider this scene. You have a back injury. You are in pain and somewhat depressed. You've been sitting in a wheelchair and waiting for hours in the rehabilitation area. Finally someone with an annoyed look comes over, towers over you, and between chews of gum starts telling you what to do to move to a standing position. You try it and in an exasperated tone the person says, "No, that isn't what I said to do. Use your legs!" You try again. But when you look up at the therapist to see if you are doing it correctly, he or she is looking across the room, paying no attention to you. Would you feel confident that he or she cared if you got better? Of course not.

With almost no extra effort or time, that same therapist can have a dramatic impact on how a patient responds to the prescribed treatment. Replay the scene. Only this time, the therapist approaches you with a smile. As he sits down beside you he establishes good eye contact as he says, "Hello Mrs. Smith. I'm Jim Jones, your physical therapist. Today I will be assisting you in learning how to easily get up from a sitting position without hurting your back."

After demonstrating the proper procedure, he smiles directly at you, touches your arm and asks if you understand how to stand up. He then firmly encourages you to try it. As you start to rise, he talks you through each movement with an enthusiastic voice, correcting you with encouragement when you make a wrong movement and congratulating you when you are standing. Wouldn't you respond better to this therapist than the first one? Of course.

The difference in the two are not just in what he said verbally such as calling you by name and stating his own name, occupation and a specific goal, but also by his facial expression and encouraging tone of voice. By sitting down to make eye contact and touching your arm, he established a feeling of caring and working together to accomplish the goal.

Each patient comes to your service with different health, personal, and psychological needs. They often come with specific expectations and even prejudices. These factors plus age, economic level, and education all precondition a person to accept—or reject—your help. For example, if you are working primarily with people over 40, obvious tattoos or multiple body piercings may make them reject you. They are likely to see tattoos and unusual body piercings as major health risks and worn primarily by uneducated bikers or risk takers. They may even be afraid you contracted AIDS or hepatitis from the needles. They may ask themselves, "Will this person who risks their health, take a risk with mine?" The moral of this example is to avoid any blatant appearance of tattoos that may create a barrier with your patients. If you chose to be tattooed, I strongly suggest that you select a body site that is easily hidden by your clothes.

Use this as a rule for wearing your non-verbal messages: When in doubt or uncertain if a body adornment, garment, accessory, hair style, or scent is appropriate for work—don't wear it!

Looking Professional

Appropriate is a key word in developing an effective professional image. Your appearance and attire needs to be appropriate for both the type of facility and the type of patient you will be assisting.

Guidelines

When in doubt about what is appropriate for any new job or clinical experience, ask. Most institutions do have guidelines as to what attire is preferred and what is inappropriate for the types of care provided and patients' expectations. In some health care facilities, uniforms may be required, while in others scrubs may be an option. In many, street clothes are the norm. Your choices of the style, color, fit, fabric, prints, and accessories even for scrubs will send a message that says "professional" or not. Your personal grooming will also add or detract from your image. Here are some tips for making appropriate choices that will help you develop a totally professional appearance.

Grooming

Clean. Looking squeaky clean from hair to shoes is a must. Tidy, under control hair is more professional than long flowing locks. Nails should be smoothly manicured (no chipped polish) and short enough to eliminate scratching any patient. Shoes should be polished and replaced at the first signs of wear. Garments should be spotless and pressed (at least when you arrive!). A strong scent of any kind can have a negative effect. A body free of unpleasant odors, with a hint of subtle fragrance or aftershave scents, plus fresh breath is always acceptable.

Posture

Good posture telegraphs self-confidence. Stand tall, throw those shoulders back, tuck that tummy in, take a deep breath, and smile. You will look capable and confident.

Apparel

Whether you wear scrubs, a uniform, or your own clothing, consider wearing a lab coat over them. The medical lab coat has the same effect as a suit jacket in a corporation. It instantly communicates that you are professional.

While psychiatric units may eliminate last names from your name tag for safety reasons, when possible wear a full name tag with your profession or specialty clearly stated in large letters that can easily be read from a distance and by the elderly. Example:

Pat Bradley, MS, OTR/L
OCCUPATIONAL THERAPY

Legible name tags let the public and other staff members know who you are and what you do. Otherwise, expect everyone to address every health care professional as, "Hey nurse".

Today, the public is truly in the dark about who does what for them. In years past the white cap with a black band made it very clear to patients who was a registered nurse. During a recent stay in a hospital my caregivers were a mystery to me. There were no visual clues to help me distinguish the supervising nurse from the cleaning staff, nor the attending physician from a nurse's aide. Patients need to know who you are. Wear your credentials, pins, and badges—you've worked hard for them. Wear them with pride.

Investing in a professional looking wardrobe pays off. Here are guidelines to assist you in making wise wardrobe choices.

Styles

Figures come in all sizes, shapes, and weights. Regardless of your figure challenges, you can choose garments that will minimize any weight or appearance problems and emphasize your best features. While the scope of this chapter limits the amount of specific guidelines that

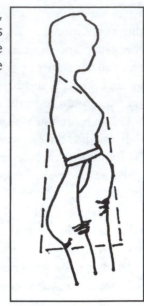

Figure 5-3. Long, loose, unstructured tops and jackets that hang straight from the shoulders can hide many figure problems.

can be included, here are some general hints that will assist you in making decisions (Larkey, 1991).

OUTSIDE AND INSIDE LINES

The silhouette of a garment can reveal or conceal the silhouette of your body (Figures 5-3 and 5-4).

HORIZONTAL AND VERTICAL LINES

Understanding the impact of the direction of a line within a garment will help you create flattering illusions. Study the rectangles in Figure 5-5.

Both rectangles are exactly the same size. Notice, however, that the one with the vertical line appears taller, while the one with the horizontal line looks wider (Figure 5-6). (Tip: Wear *vertical* lines on the parts of your body you want to lengthen or narrow. Wear *horizontal* lines on the part of your body you want to widen or shorten.)

NECKLINES

If you tend to gain weight in the facial area or have a round shaped face or broad jawline, be aware of this concept: Repeating a shape will emphasize it. Compare the two face shapes in Figure 5-7. They are exactly the same width (if you doubt it, measure them). (Tip: An open neckline opens communication between people. It makes you look friendlier. If you need a power look as an administrator or a presenter at a conference, button up.)

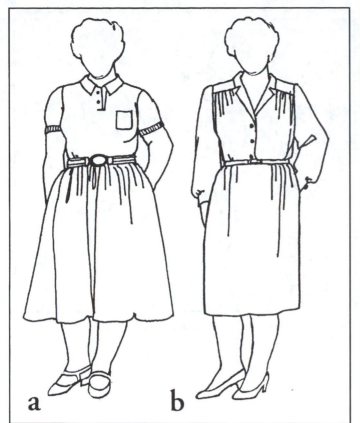

Figure 5-4. a. Reveals. (High collar shortens neck, tight top with breast pocket and short sleeves emphasize full bosom, belt accents a wide waist, full gathered skirt adds volume to full hips, shoes with straps shorten her legs.) b. Conceals. A slimmer and more professional looking woman. (Looser silhouette hides extra curves, fuller top with gathered yoke allows room for bosom, straighter skirt slims hips, low shoes elongate legs.)

Shoulder Lines

If you are petite, short, or round shouldered, wearing shoulder pads that square up your shoulders will add an aura of authority and credibility. Others will take you more seriously. If you have wide hips, extending your shoulders with pads will visually balance your lower body. If you have heavy shoulders or arms, add a thin shoulder pad with a blunt edge to create the illusion of a corner rather than a curve. You'll look slimmer.

Fit

Ease of wear is very important in the health care professions. Garments should be large enough to be unrestrictive without looking sloppy. Too tight, and you will

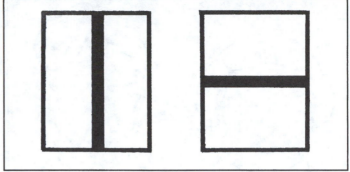

Figure 5-5. Vertical and horizontal lines.

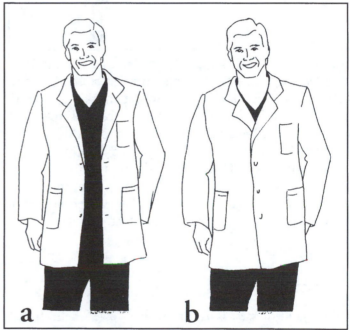

Figure 5-6. In the drawings above, when the lab coat is worn open: a. the two vertical lines make you look up and down the body, creating the illusion of a tall, slim body. When the coat is closed b. your eye follows the horizontal hemline across the body—especially if the jacket and lower garment are different colors. Place horizontal lines carefully on your body—they widen or shorten the figure.

look like you are gaining weight. Revealing your bosom, bulging biceps, upper arms, or thighs sends too sensuous a message for a professional image.

Men's trousers worn too loose and baggy or precariously low may require unprofessional "hitching" motions to keep them on. Low slung pants also create the illusion that a man's legs are short and stubby.

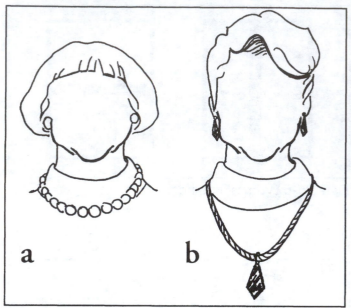

Figure 5-7. a. Full bangs create a horizontal line that widens and shortens the face, adding volume to a full face. The repetitions of a round neckline, round beads, and a round face make her face look fuller. b. Hair that is flatter on the sides creates a vertical shape that thins the face. Half-bangs and height on the crown add to this illusion. By adding a visually dominant necklace that creates a V-shape, the impact of the round neckline is minimized. The V-neckline of a lab coat would create the same effect.

FIT TESTS

Tops and dresses: Raise arms; then lower them. If the garment gets "stuck" on any part of you, try the next size. As manufacturers do not label all sizes exactly the same way, the size number on the tag is not as important as the way you look in the garment. A larger size that fits with ease will actually make you look slimmer. Cut the size tag out if the number on it bothers you!

FITTING SLACKS AND SKIRTS

Check size by sitting down and then standing up. Does the garment bind across your legs as you sit? Are major wrinkles evident across the abdomen or hip joint when you stand? Bend over and squat as you would in assisting a patient. Are seams straining? Does your shirt tail pull out? Are your slacks so baggy or riding so low as to threaten a "mooning" incident? If so, buy a size that fits better (Figure 5-8).

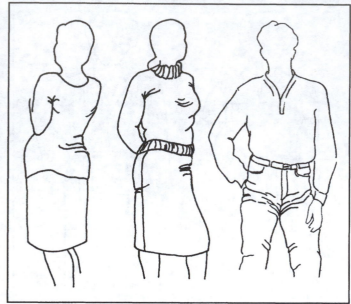

Figure 5-8. Wrinkles create horizontal lines.

Fabric

The crispness or draping properties of a fabric also affect how your body is camouflaged or revealed. *Knit fabrics reveal*, especially when a knit top is worn over knit pants. Every time you raise your arms, your top or jacket will ride up—but not down—because knit-nap sticks together. You will have to constantly pull your top down. Crisp, medium-weight, smooth woven fabrics conceal and slide up and down with ease.

Fabric bulk: Avoid wearing thick, bulky fabrics where you are "bulky". Example: If you are top-heavy combine a lightweight top with a heavier weight pant or skirt. This will help visually balance your body (Figure 5-9).

Prints, Size and Spacing

Many uniforms and scrubs now come in a variety of prints. What print size will flatter you?

Large people should avoid large prints, true or false?

I hope you answered false, because large people can wear large prints. Look at a print and notice if the shapes "bump" into each other or overlap. It is the space between the shapes that will make a body appear larger, not the actual size of the shapes. Figure 5-10 shows the same style made up in three types of floral prints. Notice how the eye follows the line of flowers in A, while it moves across the

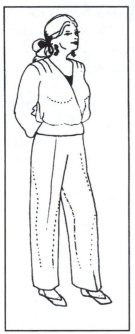

Figure 5-9. A loose surplice-styled top worn with straight-leg slacks creates better visual balance for a heavy upper torso than a bulky top with tight pants!

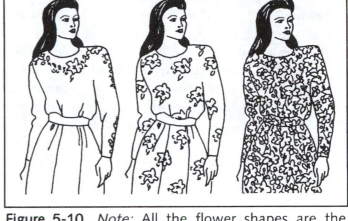

Figure 5-10. *Note:* All the flower shapes are the same size.

body (connecting the dots) in B, and then in C you see the whole garment at once. If you are large, choose A or C.

Color

Color is critical in helping you appear healthy and glowing. If you hear how tired, rather than how terrific, you look, it is probably the lack of flattering colors and/or makeup. Color has a stronger visual impact than clothing styles. It is what others will notice first about you. A drab or draining color can make you look worse than your patients.

Not every color looks good on every person, and not every person looks equally good in every color. To identify the colors that flatter you, look first at the colors above your neck—the colors you never take off—your skin tone, and hair color. More than your height or weight, your body colors are the key to selecting the color intensity and print size that will enhance you.

Consider how some cultures have developed traditional clothing that reflects their physical characteristics. Over centuries, their choices of flattering colors and print sizes have become established as preferred attire. For example, envision Hawaiians who typically have black hair and bronzed skin.

Q. What types of colors and prints do they wear?
A. Intense, bright, vivid or dark colors in bold patterns.

Now envision a man or woman from England with fair skin and light brown or auburn hair.

Q. What range of colors and prints do they typically wear?
A. Soft, subdued colors in small florals, glen plaids, or tweeds.

Now switch their clothes. Envision the tall, fair, British person in a big vivid Hawaiian printed shirt or muumuu. Put the Hawaiian in an English tweed suit. Both would be a visual disaster. The English person would be overwhelmed and the Hawaiian would look washed out. Why? Because their clothing colors do not relate to their body colors.

(Tip: The stronger your body colors (skin and hair), the brighter your wardrobe colors should be and the larger and bolder your prints may be. The softer and more blended your skin and hair color combination, the softer and more blended your wardrobe colors and prints should be.)

Buying clothing in the same brightness will also coordinate your purchases, thus saving you money. Brights mix easily with brights; medium brights with medium brights; and subdued colors with other subdued colors. What fails to mix or match are wardrobes that include bright, medium bright, subdued, and drab colors. (Tip: Drab, dirty-looking colors do not make any person look healthy.)

If people often ask you if you feel okay or remark on how tired you look, it may be because you have to wear stark "nurse's white." It can make some people look exhausted—before they start their shift.

Q. What can you do to keep from looking drained or exhausted if you are required to wear pure white?

A. Add a softer color near your face.

If allowed, add a colorful crew or turtle neck top under a white scrub suit or lab coat. Or layer a colorful vest or sweater over a uniform. If the dress code at your facility does not allow additional colored garments, use your accessories to introduce color. For women, a touch of color with makeup, earrings or a hair ornament can soften "wipe-out white". A hint of natural cheek color on glasses will make both men and women look healthier. Tints on lenses can easily be added, changed, or adjusted on your existing glasses by an eyeglass specialist. (Tip: Adding a hint of natural blush color at the bottom of glasses will make you look healthy.)

If you can wear regular clothing to work, follow this tip to mixing separates. Each time you buy a lower garment, buy a matching accessory to wear near your face. Example: Combine dark green slacks with a peach colored top, then pull your hair back with a dark green scrunchie. You'll look wonderfully coordinated. (Tip: To coordinate colorful separates, repeat near your face the color you are wearing below your waist.)

Since the goal is to send a message to your boss, your peers, and your patients that you are a competent, healthy, health care professional, it is vital to determine if your image sends this message. Every aspect of your image from hairstyle to shoe style, attitude, posture, and facial expression contributes—or detracts—from a professional look. To evaluate what message your own image is sending and to see yourself as objectively as others do, test your image impact every time you get dressed by doing the Blink Test.

The Blink Test

Here is how to see your "instant impression" very objectively.

1. Stand 5 or more feet away from a full length mirror.
2. Close your eyes. (It won't work unless you do.)
3. Open. Instantly—what do you see first?

Do you look totally coordinated from head to toe? Do you look professional? If your eyes go instantly to one item, it is what others will notice first too. If any part of your appearance strikes a jarring note when you open

your eyes, like the business women who wear athletic shoes with their power suits, change it. Repeat the Blink Test, making changes until all the parts of your apparel are sending the same message—I am a competent health care professional.

Too often we send "mixed messages." A uniform worn with large dangling earrings and multicolored fingernails won't pass the professional Blink Test; nor will wearing professional attire one day and the next day deciding to wear something that expresses what a fun-loving party animal you really are. Be smart. Save your personal clothing statements for your social life.

Your career requires that you look professional on the job. This is not to say that you cannot add a touch of personality with accessories, print choices, and even your favorite colors. Just keep this question in mind each time you get dressed for work, "Will my appearance today help my patients have confidence in me and my ability to help them?" I hope the answer is "Yes" every time you go to work.

References

Cash, T. F. (1990). The psychology of physical appearance: Aesthetics, attributes, and images. In *Body Images*. New York, NY: The Guilford Press. (pp. 71-72).

Fleschner, M. (1995). Power talk. *Personal Selling Power*, (July/August, pp. 13-18).

Larkey, J. (1991). *Flatter your figure*. New York, NY: Simon and Schuster.

Mehrabian, A. (1981). *Silent messages*. Belmont, CA: Wadsworth Publishing.

Thourlby, W. (1978). *You are what you wear*. New York, NY: Signet, The New American Library, Inc.

The illustrations for this chapter are from the *Flatter Your Figure* book, and are used with permission from Simon & Schuster and Jan Larkey. For additional information or seminars, write Jan Larkey, 126 Hawthorn Street, Pittsburgh, PA, 15218; or fax (412) 244-0431.

Exercises for Professional Presentation

1. List five positive, non-verbal clues you can use to communicate better with your patients.

   1. _____   4. _____

   2. _____   5. _____

   3. _____

2. List five negative, non-verbal clues that may hinder your effectiveness with patients.

   1. _____   4. _____

   2. _____   5. _____

   3. _____

3. List a person from any occupation (or a character in a movie, book, or story) whose change in appearance had a positive or adverse effect on the goal of that person. What did they change? What impact did it have? Discuss your answers.

4. Break into groups. Each group should develop a dress code for a specific situation. Determine the following job description:

Type of health care professional:

Position held:

Type of facility:

Ages of patients:

Type of care given by the professional:

Physical activity required by the professional:

Develop a professional dress code for the job described above using the chart below:

	Male	Female
Grooming:		
Hair style		
Facial hair		
Nails		
Apparel:		
Styles		
Colors		
Accessories		
Shoes		

Check all the types/styles of clothing, body adornment, or habits that are NOT appropriate for the job described above. Add others.

	Male	Female
Jeans		
Sweats		
Stirrup pants		
Shorts		
Tank tops		
Open toe shoes		
Tennis type shoes		
Fragrances		
Tattoos		
Jewelry on hands		
Gum chewing		
Exposed upper arms		
Exposed thighs		
Dangle earrings		
Multiple earrings		
Nail polish		

Chapter Six

Initiative

Threese A. Clark, MS, OTR/L

Initiative: Changing possible to probable success

Skill + Knowledge + Common Sense + Emotional Maturity + Opportunity = **Possible** Success

Skill + Knowledge + Common Sense + Emotional Maturity + Opportunity + INITIATIVE = **Probable** Success

Hey, Joe! I just met your new Coordinator of Student Internships. What a ball of fire that gal is. She certainly appears to be both self-directed and a self-starter. Rumor has it that student and supervisor morale has already taken a turn for the better. She's what the Old Man use to call a "go-getter". Watch yourself. She'll be taking over your job as Supervisor before you know it.

The above example of an informal workplace conversation, or its equivalent, might occur when someone recognizes an individual who they feel, or fear, has the characteristics that promote career growth and advancement. Those characteristics and that potential can be present in a janitor or a brain surgeon. It is not the level of the endeavor but rather the manner in which it is accomplished that makes the difference and accounts for the success or failure of the venture. Although characteristics such as skill, knowledge, common sense, and emotional maturity in the presence of opportunity may assist with the accomplishment of personal and professional goals and success, they alone are not sufficient to guarantee it. Motivation and initiative are the workhorses that deliver. Success in any task is a ladder that cannot be climbed with your hands in your pockets.

What are initiative and motivation? What effect do initiative and motivation have on personal success and life satisfaction? What is the connection between personal success and professional advancement? How does the personal success of an occupation's practitioners translate into the advancement and success of the profession as a whole? The following pages will attempt to answer these questions.

Definitions

Definitions (as found in *Webster's New World Dictionary*, 1995 edition):

Initiative - readiness to attempt or engage in what requires energy or daring: enterprise; ambition; drive; push

Motivation - something that rouses the mind or spirits or incites to activity: stimulus; catalyst; impetus; impulse; incentive; incitation; incitement; instigation; propellant; provocative; push; spur; stimulant

Initiative and motivation are words often used interchangeably. However, these definitions suggest that initiative is an innate characteristic, while motivation is external. Still, the two are often observed working in close proximity and are difficult to separate. While initiative may be an internal force, it takes motivation to turn it into overt action. Without motivation, initiative may never be exercised. We may not be able to instill initiative in ourselves or another individual, but we can motivate, incite, or stimulate it. The outward evidence of successful motivation and the subsequent use of initiative is action. Action, therefore, is the desired personal or professional response that is the end product of initiative. Action supports personal achievement and research, treatment or intervention processes, personal and professional growth, adaptation to change, and ultimately, the success and survival of an individual, an occupation or a profession. It is our responsibility, whatever our role (student, clinician, educator, role model, or mentor), to motivate and therefore encourage, develop, enhance, expand, or otherwise awaken initiative in ourselves and in those with whom we interact. Dreaming without action, questioning without engagement, or wanting without doing does not generate accomplishment. For the purpose of this discussion, motivation and initiative will be considered as an essential couple, both necessary to obtain the desired result. The term "man" throughout this narrative refers to "humankind" and does not refer to gender. Also, the use of the word "individual" is meant to refer to oneself as well as to others.

Motivation (initiative) is a dream that put on workclothes.

Erma Bombeck (1996) once proposed that initiative is the talent to recognize what you have going for you and to use it to its fullest. I would further suggest that initiative is not only the recognition of what you have going for you, but also the courage to see what may not be advantageous and to act to change it. It is this behavior that we need to nurture. We must provide or create a climate within which it is safe to risk personal and professional inspection and which fosters the shift from thought to the action that is the agent of change and growth. In encouraging and supporting others, we ourselves benefit. By attempting to motivate others, we find ourselves encouraged and motivated. Practice with motivating others improves our own initiative and motivation and moves us from a novice to the experienced and competent professional/practitioner.

The motivated individual, the individual who is taking initiative, was described at the beginning of this chapter as self-directed — as a "ball of fire", a "self-starter", or a "go-getter". He or she has personal power. Power that enables him or her to adapt and change, to grow and improve. Where does this initiative, this personal power come from? Is it a trait inherited at birth? Does it reside on one of the chromosomes or in a DNA pattern? If it did, we could not hope to influence it.

Significance

Initiative is the act of taking control and exercising ownership of one's actions. It is the freedom to choose to perform and therefore, comes from within. We cannot control the inner drives and attitudes of an individual. We can, however, motivate the individual to question or examine his or her beliefs, attitudes, opinions, actions, and values by providing a climate in which acceptance and unconditional encouragement supports such examination. This is not to suggest that we accept inappropriate or potentially harmful behaviors or actions, but that we assist the individual with recognizing these for him- or herself and offer support for correction or change. In this manner, we create an individual who can become more independent in these pursuits and who may become the master professional/practitioner or professional leader who contributes to the growth and advancement of a profession/occupation as a whole. However, if not the master or leader, individuals can still be instrumental in influencing, for better or worse, each person (client, coworker, neighbor, etc.) with whom they interact during their lifetime and/or career.

Background

A belief generally shared by numerous professionals states that man's basic nature is to act, rather than to be acted upon (Covey, 1989). The social sciences and occupational science embrace the concept of "man as an active being" and the belief that "purposeful activity allows man to adapt and change." Implied in the belief that man is an active being is the idea of choice. Choice gives man the ability to exert a degree of control over his or her circumstances and environment. It is this ability to exert control upon and to influence one's life that health care professionals use as a tool to assist themselves and the individuals they serve to prevent, control and/or adapt to the changes that are inevitable throughout the life span. As we strive to understand ourselves and our clients from a holistic arena, we gather and appraise information on values, priorities, experiences, and life stories. Through this activity it becomes evident that people do not react to situations and circumstances with identical responses. Based on life experiences, resources, strengths, cultural background, religious convictions, socioeconomic status, etc., choice becomes a very personal phenomenon. Initiative and motivation are strongly influenced by choice and a conviction that we have a choice — a certainty that man can influence his own life and that we are not at the mercy of pure fate. Man chooses which circumstances to respond to, and (within certain parameters) what that response will be. As the ability to improve, expand, or augment choice can be enhanced through learning, so can initiative or motivation be affected. Conversely, the ability to choose which circumstances to respond to empowers us to create circumstances. Life and learning is developmental. Present circumstance is the child of the past and the parent of the future.

What in the nature of man supports the development of initiative? What actions and environment will motivate an individual to tap his capabilities? During the 1960s and 70s a great deal of energy was expended by individuals to "find and understand themselves." What was the underlying motivation that ignited this search? Maslow felt that man had a need to discover and make the best use of his talent (Carr-Ruffino, 1993), while Childs believed that it was inner drives and impulses that caused a person to act in a particular way to ensure the satisfaction of his needs (Coombs, 1991).

However, satisfied or balanced needs do not motivate. Man is in a constant cycle of balance and imbalance. Man is motivated to seek and strive for balance. The search for balance leads to action. Action leads to change, adaptation, and learning. Once the lower level needs for survival and safety are met, man can pursue the higher level need for self-actualization. Movement to self-actualization requires initiative, motivation, and risk. It requires the challenging of habits, as well as the questioning of internalized principles and patterns of behaviors (Covey, 1989). Movement occurs at the intersection of knowledge (the what and why of theory), skill (the how to), and desire (the initiative/motivation).

Extrinsic vs. Intrinsic Initiative/Motivation

There are two distinctive forms of initiative/motivation. Extrinsic, or basic, initiative/motivation is based on the requirements of others (Entwistle, 1988). It is the level of initiative/motivation common to the novice learner or young professional/practitioner who is driven by a fear of failure, the need for professional status, or a desire to belong. It does not produce a long-lasting effect. The learner who studies to please the professor or his or her parents comes to mind. Remove the power of a grade and/or the need for financial support and the "motivation" to study disappears and the material "learned" may be forgotten.

This now is the basic level of initiative/motivation and is externally oriented. Man is influenced to varying degrees by socially acquired motivators such as the need for affiliation, for power, and for achievement. Learning at this level is influenced by the expectation of a reward (Carr-Ruffino, 1993).

The rewards in the area of affiliation affect the quantity, if not the quality, of relationships. The individual seeks a sense of belonging, recognition, or group cohesion—often joining multiple groups or organizations. The feedback and communication obtained from these affiliations are the vehicles by which success is measured and evaluated. The reward in the arena of power is control. A person may seek to control others or to control events. Control decreases the uncomfortable or unknown and gives a feeling of security. A reward for achievement may also be a feeling of security, a belief that a new skill or more knowledge will allow one the material benefits that will ensure success, safety, acceptance, and so on. These rewards are often in the form of titles, money, or position. Our society appears to be rather advanced at stimulating this level of initiative/motivation. We set educational requirements, establish pay scales based on job responsibilities or skills, reward power and control with titles and position, institute price structures for needed or desired commodities, and create sets of perceived needs. While this may result in temporary satisfaction, security, or commitment, it does not result in long-term fulfillment. The learner does and will mature. His values will change and he will become increasingly discontented. Lacking the deeper level of internal initiative/motivation, he may not even realize the source of his dissatisfaction and restlessness, doomed to seek more of the very things that have become unfulfilling.

On the other hand, intrinsic motivation/initiative is derived from personal understanding and development and provides a stage for continued life-long accomplishment. It is from the development of motivation/initiative that is internally fueled that the ability to achieve lasting satisfaction is born. This internally fueled motivation/initiative will ensure life-long learning. It is, however, more difficult to foster and encourage.

Intrinsic motivators include a hope for success, academic interest, the search for autonomy and internal control, the wish to have control over personal resources and talents and the desire to make a personal contribution (Coombs, 1991; Covey, 1991; Entwistle, 1988). Intrinsic motivation/initiative is process- not product-oriented. Work or study is viewed as a process through which one reaches an end, not as a worthwhile end in itself. The individual is committed to the goal rather than to the method of achieving it (Carr-Ruffino, 1993). The challenge is to improve and contribute (Wacks, 1993). The student who has internalized a desire for life-long learning as a means to improve his or her own life and the lives of others will not be affected by the removal of external rewards. The acquiring of knowledge becomes the process through which to experience achievement and contribute to society. The learner who has achieved this level is a challenge to his or her professors, mentors, friends, and colleagues. They are the individuals that we must run to keep up with and who challenge us to explore, expand, and grow with them.

Intrinsic initiative/motivation is the level we wish to develop — the level which, while providing the foundation for personal achievement, will also ensure the growth of the individual, an occupation, a profession, or society as a whole. What are the essentials necessary for this development? What basic characteristics do we look for and then strive to advance and promote?

Development of Initiative/Motivation

As the child learning to stand first holds on to his mother's knee, so does the learner hold on to his or her teachers or mentors, proven facts, and tested ideas. With encouragement and the right motivators, the child moves farther from that supporting knee, backing away to arm's length and finally daring to let go. So must we move ourselves and others developmentally through the need for support and encouragement into the universe of self-awareness, independent will, holistic conscious ness, and unbridled imagination. These things will promote competency and self-fulfillment, while advancing society and our knowledge of man. This requires risk not only for the learner but for the educator, mentor, friend, family member(s), or colleague(s) involved with the person. We must move away from the formal approach of teaching and learning facts and techniques — trusting ourselves to acquire these as a

consequence of learning — to a proactive model of advocating problem-centered, logically-structured thinking. Thinking that promotes and is promoted by action is the end product of initiative/motivation. As students and learners we must not demand complete provision of all facts or work for grades or extrinsic reward alone but must embrace process over product. We must stretch to challenge ourselves to step beyond our comfort zone and explore the unknown or next level of knowing. The external reward will follow. A learner who studies to understand a concept, technique, theory, or process will find that the grade/reward or clinical/professional success will be there. The individual who learns material for the grade/reward may not find success in clinical/professional work as he or she is not able to use or has forgotten the concept, technique, theory, or process. He or she is often unable to draw upon past learning to solve present problems.

The outward manifestation of initiative/motivation is a level of energy, enthusiasm, and determination that indicates the individual is serious about the activity in which he or she is engaged and which suggests an acceptance of responsibility for the outcome. The motivated person appears to have a sense of the larger picture and his or her position within it. He or she is proactive, begins with the end in mind, and is able to set priorities or "put first things first" (Covey, 1989). Generally the older, mature individual who has a measure of control over his or her life and is relatively free from major life stressors participates more fully and for longer periods of time in the practice of higher level intrinsic motivation. He or she appears to possess a focused awareness to enjoy and find pleasure in the activity. The ability to engage in motivated behaviors changes with both age and life circumstances. It is our challenge as learners, educators, mentors, and role models to encourage and develop these behaviors in our students, colleagues, and associates, as well as in ourselves.

Progress always involves risk; You can't steal second base and keep your foot on first.
Frederick Wilcox (Kaplan and Kaplan, 1982)

Impractical observers often describe the self-motivated as competent individuals who appear to be better than average at making "good" or "right" choices. The better an individual knows himself and the more faithful he is to that knowledge, the more chance for success his choices possess. Basic learning, that reproduction of a body of knowledge, is therefore not enough. We must do more than teach and learn facts. We must go beyond the surface and be concerned with more than task completion. It is the personal understanding of formal knowledge, and the internalization of essential principles and incidentals that allow the learner to extract meaning from learning. Meaning that will promote life success. It is this deeper learning that allows the individual to develop the confidence to challenge ideas and today's evidence or facts. This allows for the formation of questions and arguments that will confirm, refute, refine, or advance our body of both formal and personal knowledge. It is this holistic learning that will advance and elevate our lives, our profession, and our world and motivate us to even loftier heights. Our challenge is to find both the internal initiative and the external motivators in ourselves and others that will ensure the continued growth and development of knowledge and of mankind. We must meet individuals on their level and provide opportunities for growth. The idea of "right" and "wrong" answers must be replaced with opportunities to find the "best" answer given the situation and its contextual parameters. The learner's answer must be accepted as correct given his or her present knowledge and experience. Growth and the formation of better answers comes from challenging with additional information or the provision of advanced experiences. We must reward all attempts and provide opportunity for safe risk-taking. Conversely, learners must be open to "best" answer rather than to "right" answer learning, and must understand that with the acquisition of additional knowledge and skill, the best answer may change. Success stimulates growth and advanced risk-taking behaviors. This is the substance of initiative/motivation.

Additionally, success in developing internal initiative/motivation results in increased self and life satisfaction. This satisfaction is the parent of personal autonomy and responsibility. These traits not only benefit the individual, but benefit the profession through increased job satisfaction, increased morale, and increased self-assurance. These traits impart the courage to think independently and question theory and application. The acts of thinking and questioning may result in improved professional/occupational standards of care, development of innovative intervention approaches, more complete data gathering leading to improved intervention planning and goal setting, better understanding of an individual's values, objectives and priorities, and a willingness to evaluate outcomes. They impart the ability to challenge the status quo and enable man to strive to contribute and improve. Only persons possessing motivation/initiative reach this level.

Therefore, individuals must be proactive and strive to develop these attributes.

The more chance there is of stubbing your toe, the more chance you have of stepping into success. (Author Unknown)

A proactive model for learning requires the presentation of a stimulus. The stimulus must not demand a specific or predetermined response but should impart a freedom of choice. The response that develops should be immediately evaluated and feedback offered in a problem-solving approach. The feedback should be specific, identifiable, easily digested, and should reward the risk(s) taken by the learner. This approach to learning must identify the behaviors to be rewarded, reward those behaviors immediately and specifically, offer the reward consistently, and ensure that the offered reward has value and meaning for the recipient (i.e., the reward must be worth the risk). The mentor must be able to communicate his belief in both the ability of the learner to perform the task successfully, and in the fact that the effort will result in a desired outcome. An understanding of the requirements and expectations of the exercise by both the mentor and learner is essential. Attachment of the experience to the real world is advantageous.

This approach fosters risk-taking and rewards an individual's attempts to take responsibility for his or her own learning. It rewards initiative and motivates the learner to take the next step or to risk again.

It is desirable for both parties in a learning experience to be active participants. The mentor should offer limited direction, unconditional support, and timely, sensitive feedback. It is important to safeguard the learner's self-esteem while challenging him to greater achievement. Solutions should not be given and assistance should be offered only upon request, and only then in a problem-solving fashion. The mentor should be skillful in active listening and be capable of responding with empathy. Assistance must be given without taking responsibility for the outcome. Consistent, constructive feedback is essential. Success must be measured by set criteria and not be competitive in nature. The individual must understand and embrace this learning approach. He or she must request information or assistance in a manner compatible with this approach and move beyond the idea that the mentor will furnish the knowledge or answer. The learner must also accept responsibility for his or her learning and view the process as a partnership.

Learning is based in part on a belief that every person has an equal chance to become better than he is and that learning is the vehicle through which that chance is actualized. If every person has an equal chance to become better, what is the roadblock that prevents this from happening? Opportunity, whether lost, missed, misunderstood, or never given, may well be the answer to the puzzle. It is our responsibility as individuals, educators, parents, mentors, friends, and citizens of the world to offer or request these opportunities whenever and however an occasion to do so presents itself.

Educational research also suggests that man learns faster from success than from failure (Covey, 1990). Therefore, we must provide the required amount of direction, knowledge, resources, and support to ensure that success. As a learner, we must request only the amount of assistance necessary and be accountable for our own successes or failures. As mentors we must coach without rescuing and link accomplishment to action. Teaching should be informal and assigned tasks open-ended. To develop self-motivation/initiative the learner must experience an ever-decreasing need to depend on the educator or mentor and should be given ample time to accomplish the task goal. Interpretative assessment with feedback is essential.

Methods and Ideas

The average learner is not ready to jump into this approach. he or she has been educated in an essentially formal manner and feel insecure and fearful when that structure is removed. They may demand a formal presentation of fact and may become angry if that approach is not the largest percent of their learning experience. Both planned and unplanned opportunities to promote independent learning and critical problem-solving will need to be carefully integrated into the learning experience. The mentor will need to be ever-vigilant, watching for every and all opportunities to reward those behaviors that can be built upon and used to enhance initiative/motivation. Individual learners must be open to a new approach. These opportunities may be as simple as reading a portion of a well-written document to colleagues or asking the learner's permission to use his or her work as an example for future discussion, or it may be as complicated as assisting an individual with getting deserving work published. Incorporating learner ideas and/or suggestions into experiences, processes or procedures, and giving credit to the individual for that idea or suggestion not only encourages that person but may motivate others to emulate the

rewarded behavior. Each time a risk results in a reward, or at least does not produce a punishment, it makes the next risk a little easier to take. Sharing personal stories of failure and success is also helpful. Humanizing the perceived expert puts the goal of competence within the realm of the possible to achieve. Encouraging the individual to laugh at himself and keep in perspective his or her less than successful attempts at being the model professional or practitioner goes a long way toward enabling repeated attempts. It is those repeated attempts that are important. After all, practice makes perfect!

Life stories, self-assessments, or case studies/grand rounds are flexible and open-ended methods for a more planned approach to the development of initiative/motivation. The learner is encouraged to develop an entire life story for an individual or themselves, or to analyze a specific case. He or she is rewarded for the completeness and resourcefulness of his or her analysis. Groups of learners are then given the same life story or case summary and a life problem is introduced or identified. The groups are allowed to solve the problem in any manner that they feel meets the criteria established. In most instances one or more solutions, which will differ from group to group, will evolve. A debate between groups with opposing solutions is held, with the remaining groups offering feedback on the effectiveness of the defense and reasoning used. In this manner the learners are exposed to numerous approaches and solutions to a common problem. Critical thinking skills are challenged and initiative/motivation is rewarded. Clinical problem-solving task groups and preceptor/mentor programs are another approach that can be invaluable in promoting and developing self-directed behaviors.

Developing a Rubric that divides goals, aspirations, and behaviors into levels of achievement can be helpful in assessing where an individual is and defining what behaviors must be present to advance. For example, an individual expresses a wish to move into supervision. He or she develops a Rubric that defines the behaviors he or she observes in individuals at the various job performance levels within his or her organization (entry level staff, intermediate level practitioner/professional, advanced/respected practitioner/professional, and management). He or she determines which level he or she is functioning within and sets out to achieve those behaviors that are present in the level that he or she aspires to but does not now possess.

Finally, individuals can learn and use various tools and/or diagrams to direct their own learning or to solve individual or group problems or concerns. These tools can act both as

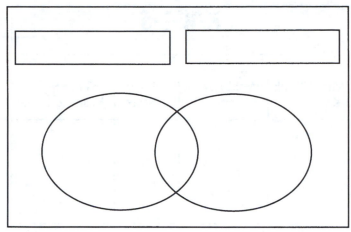

Figure 6-1. Venn Diagram.

an aid in identifying areas and opportunities for improvement, or a map or plan to achieve a goal. One example of this approach is the Venn Diagram (Figure 6-1). The rectangles at the top may be filled in with traits, problem statements, or other key ideas and words as necessary. The outside circles are then filled in with facts that correspond with the rectangle on that side of the diagram. The overlapping area of the circles is either the strengths (components held by the problem and the solution) or weaknesses (missing pieces needed to solve the problem). With this information and assessment of the situation a plan to improve or solve the dilemma can be formulated.

Conclusion

The very elusiveness of initiative/motivation and of the behaviors that stimulate it presents a two-fold dilemma for the mentor and the learner.

How do we develop, enhance, or encourage initiative/ motivation? How do we measure or evaluate our success?

The rewards of success are too important to the learner individually (and professions as a whole) for the dilemmas presented to result in our failure to try. If we are suc-cessful with only a portion of our attempts, the results of those successes to the individual receiving services, to society as a whole, or to a profession's growth and refinement will still be immeasurable and well worth the effort.

References

Bombeck, E. (1996). *Forever, Erma: best loved writing from America's favorite humorist.* Kansas City, MO: Andrews and McMeel.

Bryham, W. C., & Cop, J. (1988). *Zapp: the lightening of empowerment.* New York, NY: Forwalt Columbine.

Carr-Ruffino, N. (1993). *The promotable woman: advancing through leadership skills,* (2nd ed.). Belmont, CA: Wadsworth Publishing Co.

Coombs (1991). Motivational strategies for intensive care nurses. *Intensive Care Nursing, 7,* 114-119.

Covey, S. R. (1989). *The seven habits of highly effective people.* New York, NY: Simon & Schuster.

Covey, S. R. (1990). *Principle-centered leadership.* New York, NY: Summit Books.

Dealy, M. F., & Bass, M. (1995). Professional development: factors that motivate staff. *Nursing Management, 26(8),* 320-321.

Entwistle, N. (1988). Motivational factors in student's approaches to learning. In R. Schmeck (Ed.). *Learning strategies and learning styles.* New York, NY: Plenum Press.

Garfield, C. (1992). *Second to none: How our smartest companies put people first.* Homewood, IL: Business One Irwin.

Kaplan, M., & Kaplan, D. (1982). *Smiles, lovable, livable, laughable lines.* Atlanta, GA: Cheers.

Kelly, R., & Caplan, J. (1993). How Bell Labs creates star performers. *Harvard Business Review,* July/Aug., 128-139.

Mabbett, P. (1987). From burned out to turned on. *The Canadian Nurse,* March, 15-19.

Mangan, P. (1993). (Editorial) Strategies for motivation. *Nursing Times, 89(12).*

Murray, D. (1994). The best single tool for motivating your staff. *Medical Economics,* April, 131-138.

Wacks, J. E. (1993). Performance appraisal as a motivational tool. *AAOHN Journal, 41(12),* 599-600.

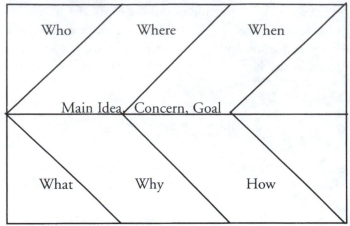

Figure 6-2. Herringbone Diagram

K-W-L-S

Topic:_____

What I Think I Know	What I Want to Know	What I Learned	What I Still Want to Know

Figure 6-3. K-W-L-S Diagram.

Exercises for Developing Initiative

1. Interview persons collecting their life stories. Describe a situation or circumstance to persons with various life stories to determine their approach to the situation. Bring the results of interviews back to class. In small groups compare the various approaches and try to determine the degree of success of the approach. Attempt to find alternatives that might have improved the outcomes.

2. Investigate personal values and beliefs. Think of a situation that occurred where you did not handle things in the manner you predicted you would. Try to determine what caused the difference between what you thought you would do or how you thought you would react and what you actually did or felt.

3. Volunteer for an assignment or experience that you are not totally comfortable with but will offer you a growth experience.

4. Form study groups that expand upon required work and offer opportunities for improvement of personal skills and knowledge.

5. Develop a Herringbone Diagram (Figure 6-2) to plan to improve a situation or to set a timeline and plan to meet a goal.

6. Using the K-W-L-S Diagram (Know, Want [to know], Learned, Still [need to know]), assess an area of knowledge or skill that you possess (Figure 6-3). Determine if you can or wish to advance this strength or if there is a weakness in performance that can be improved - fill in columns 1 and 2. Implement a plan to intervene - fill in columns 3 and 4.

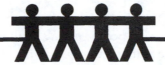

Chapter
Seven

Empathy

Marian L. Farrell, PhD, RNC

Mary E. Muscari, PhD, CRNP, CS

> The nurse sits with the woman cradling her newborn, her long-awaited first child. The woman caresses the baby's cheek and whispers, "I love you, goodbye." Tears well, but do not fall as the woman gently kisses her dead infant. The nurse touches the woman's shoulder, responding to her grief.

In the above scenario, words are unnecessary. The nurse demonstrated empathy by understanding the woman's feelings and by responding to them with her presence and the use of touch.

Empathy is the emotional and intellectual understanding of another person's feelings, thoughts, and behaviors (O'Toole, 1997). As it is a personal response to another individual, empathy involves communication within the context of relationships. In practice, empathy is the ability to relate to and understand the meaning of the experiences of another individual.

Empathy should not be confused with sympathy. Sympathy is a likeness between persons or the similarity of thoughts and feelings. With empathy, the professional understands what the client is experiencing; with sympathy, the professional shares the experience. Sympathy creates a desire to relieve suffering while empathy encourages the exploration of feelings, progressing toward problem-solving (Townsend, 1996).

The ability to empathize is affected by the professionals' own attributes, personal and professional experiences, knowledge about people, and how they themselves are feeling. The development of empathy requires that professionals get to know their clients. They need to hear their stories so that they can understand their clients' perspective. Empathetic feelings may be difficult to generate when students have no previous related experiences, and when clients are difficult to understand (Baillie, 1996). Therefore, like other professional behaviors, empathy must be nurtured through its own developmental process.

Background

Empathy is defined in the dictionary as "entering freely into another's feelings or emotions" (*World Book Dictionary*, 1968, p. 497). In 1897, Lipps introduced the term *Einfuhlung* (feeling into oneself) in his writings about aesthetic perception and appreciation. The German term was translated as empathy by Tichener in 1910 (Goldstein and Michaels, 1985, p. 4). Although Lipps is credited with defining empathy 100 years ago, the description, measurement, and development of empathy remains the focus of many researchers.

Description

Traux (1961) described empathy as involving more than just the ability of an individual to sense the needs of the other person. Empathy also involves the ability of the individual to know what the other person means. Traux described empathy as the sensitivity to the individual's current feelings and the verbal ability to communicate this understanding in a language attuned to the client's current feeling. Empathy is a term that has also been defined as the ability to perceive accurately how another person is feeling (Levenson and Reuf, 1992) and as an emotional, cognitive, communicative, and relational phenomenon (Williams, 1990).

Gladstein (1983) completed an analysis of the social and developmental psychology literature, and described empathy as a multistage interpersonal process involving emotional contagion, identification, and role-taking. He differentiated empathic responses in children from empathic responses in adolescents and adults. Goldstein and Michaels (1985) provided an extensive review of empathy, which included the following: historical and contemporary definitions, development of empathy; perceptual and affective components, the cognitive analysis, psychotherapeutic consequences, educational consequences, parenting consequences, and training.

Empathy is the ability to understand the essence of the experience of another individual. According to Jordan (1983), empathy requires a high level of psychological development and ego strength. A well-differentiated sense of self allows the individual to have a greater appreciation and sensitivity to the other individual. Within the relational framework, the sharing of life experiences provides opportunities for personal growth and a sense of connection that is essential to the development of empathy (Jordan, 1983; Surrey, 1985).

Measurement

Researchers have developed many tools to measure empathy and its constructs. Hogan (1969) developed a 64-item self-report tool to measure empathy. Grief and Hogan (1973) described characteristics of empathic persons and the use of empathy scales in research. They characterized empathic persons as being patient, affiliative, and social, with liberal, humanistic, political, and religious attitudes (Grief and Hogan, 1973). Hogan (1975) discussed the role of empathy in personality, as well as the use of an empirically-keyed empathy scale. He differentiated between trait and state empathy. Trait empathy has a genetic basis and is influenced by intelligence and early experiences. Trait empathy would be least likely to change during adulthood as a result of training. Individuals who demonstrated state empathy were more likely to change as a result of a training program.

Barrett-Lennard (1981) described a series of distinct stages that involved empathic interaction. Davis (1983)

developed the Interpersonal Reactivity Index (IRI) based upon a multidimensional approach of four areas: perspective taking, empathic concern, fantasy, and personal distress. Gagan (1983) discussed the lack of reliability of empathy measurement tools, such as the *Traux Accurate Empathy Scale* and the *Hogan's Empathy Scale*. LaMonica (1979) discussed the importance of research regarding empathy in two areas: empathy as the primary ingredient in helping process, and the relationship between empathic helpers and counseling outcome.

Growth of Empathy

Researchers have explored the development of empathy in pre-school children (Gnepp, Klayman, & Trabasso, 1982; Abraham, Kuehl, Christopherson, 1983; Freeman, 1984; Gibbs and Woll, 1985). Emde (1985) described how 2-year-old children demonstrated emotional and comforting responses to distressed individuals. Zahn-Waxler and Radke-Yarrow (1990) reviewed research of the development of empathy in young children. As a result of their review, Zahn-Waxler and Radke-Yarrow raised questions regarding earlier conceptions of young children being primarily egocentric and uncaring. They reported as early as age 2, children demonstrate the cognitive capacity to interpret the physical and psychological states of others. In addition, they found children able to demonstrate the emotional capacity necessary to affectively experience the state of others, and the behavioral repertoire to alleviate the discomfort of others. They also described how the child's temperament and environment contribute to their development of empathy.

Ungerer, Dolby, Waters, Barnette, et al. (1990) conducted a longitudinal study of 45 primiparous women and their newborns and found the presence of empathic responses in infants and young children. Fabes, Eisenberg, Karborn, Troyer, and Switzer (1994) studied the relationship between the regulation of emotional responses and comforting behaviors in children who were in kindergarten and second grade. They found that if children were able to regulate their arousal (measured by physical parameters such as heart rate), they were more likely to be empathic and not be overwhelmed by the events. Davis, Luce, and Kraus (1994) reviewed preexisting data of over 800 sets of twins to substantiate a physiological support for empathy based upon genetic predisposition. As a result of their review, they found support for the two affective facets of empathy (empathic concern and personal distress) but not the nonaffective construct of perspective-taking.

Although the development of empathy begins very early in childhood, there is a need to teach students how to continue their development of empathy, as empathy is a core attribute of health care professionals. According to Smith (1973), empathy is composed of four dimensions: rationalistic understanding, artistic understanding, practical understanding, and empirical understanding. The four dimensions serve as a philosophical framework for teaching. There is no sequencing of the four dimensions, although the four dimensions exist throughout the model. Rationalistic understanding stresses inner realities, and emotional and personally satisfying experiences. Artistic understanding describes the visual, audible, and other tangible aspects of the other person, and stresses the outer realities. Practical understanding is the degree to which one person can influence the behavior of the other individual. Empirical understanding describes the ability to predict another individual's feelings, thoughts, and behaviors.

Smith (1973) described a process for the development of empathy based upon proper planning. Smith advised the development of realistic goals that are both trainee and content centered. He encouraged frequent, precise, and objective feedback. The goals need to be sequenced to reduce stress and increase retention and use of the information. He encouraged planning to ensure that the training methods be varied and selected to achieve the goals. Teaching methods include role modeling, role playing, videotaping, and further development of communication skills. Didactic information needs to be incorporated throughout the program, particularly the clinical components. Valid criteria must be utilized in order to evaluate the success developing empathy as a result of the training program.

Evaluation needs to have both a quantitative and a qualitative component. The quantitative component can be achieved through the use of one of the many available empathy scales (following careful review of what outcomes need to be measured). Forsyth's (1980) criteria for empathy may be useful in evaluating the presence of empathy in the products of the training sessions (e.g., videotapes): consciousness of self, others, and experience; temporality (here and now, change); relationship (response, interaction, and reciprocity); accuracy; energy that varies in intensity; objectivity; validation; and freedom from judgment or evaluation. Successful training in the development of empathy is contingent upon feedback of the program outcomes to the program planners.

Presence of Empathy in Health Care Professionals

Brunt (1985) explored the effect of technology on nurses' empathy and did not find that high tech nurses had low empathic levels; rather both ICU and non-ICU nurses had only moderate empathy. "Empathy involves the process whereby helpers experience the world of their client's and then utilize those perceptions in a therapeutic manner" (Brunt, 1985, p.70). Wheeler (1988) examined the nature of empathy within Roger's systems paradigm of nursing science. She discussed clinical applications of empathy where the "nurse can facilitate the healing milieu by connecting with the patient through empathy, thus directing energy to the patient. Energy is then shared with the patient, which reestablishes the patient's own flow" (p.100).

Christiansen (1977) described use of the *Hogan Empathy Scale,* resulting in significant correlation between measured empathy and perceived ability to empathize in OT students. Wise and Page (1980) discussed the use of *Kagan's Affective Sensitivity Scale* to measure changes in empathy levels in OT students and permanent changes in empathy scores related to a group process approach.

The importance of the development of empathy has been viewed as critical to decreasing antisocial behaviors. Scavo and Buchanan (1989) described a mandatory group treatment model for male adolescent sex offenders who were in a residential treatment program. One of the focal points of the program was the development of empathic responses in the client in order to reduce antisocial behaviors. Schulman (1984) described a comprehensive theory of moral motivation designed to encompass the internalization of adult standards and the development of empathy.

Brent (1985) focused on the usefulness of empathy assessment as a strategy to assess the social functioning and possibility of psychiatric disorders in school-age children. Morgan (1983) conducted a study of school-aged children and results indicated a humanistic/psychoeducational model, utilizing the development of empathy rather than a behavioral learning model, was more effective in the interventions with emotionally disturbed children.

Developing Empathy

Empathic responses are essential within personal interactions of daily life. We all have multiple opportunities to be empathic. Here is a story from my life as an example.

Several years ago I experienced the loss of a baby. Medical professionals label this "intrauterine fetal demise." Lay persons call the experience a miscarriage. I was just starting to feel good and had adjusted to the idea of being pregnant and planning for a new baby. I went for my second prenatal visit feeling great. After a few moments of conversation, the doctor applied the Doppler so my oldest daughter and I could listen to the baby's heartbeat. Initially there was no heartbeat, and the doctor readjusted the Doppler, mumbling something about it being old. He then said that I better get an ultrasound "just to make sure everything was all right." The doctor never stated out loud what we both knew at that point — the baby was dead.

At the ultrasound department, the technician applied the ultrasound and we both saw a perfect baby with no fetal heartbeat. The technician walked out, leaving me alone in the room. He came back about 15 minutes later and said he was sorry he left. He explained that his wife had experienced a similar situation and that he felt overwhelmed and did not want to make me upset. I was left alone at a vulnerable moment because the health care provider was overwhelmed! Surely the technician felt touched, but instead of choosing an empathic response he chose to disconnect from the experience. The result for me was not only realizing that the baby was dead but also feeling abandoned. The technician was asking me at a very vulnerable point to be empathic to him, to understand why he had to leave.

The next day I was in the preoperative holding area awaiting surgery. I knew most of the nurses, orderlies, and the nurse anesthetist, but none of them came over to talk even though I was obviously crying. Fortunately one nurse walked over to me, asked what was wrong, held my hand and simply said, "I'm sorry." What a difference a little empathy can make.

In order to be empathic, one has to occasionally take the risk that the relationship will evoke strong feelings, especially if the professional experienced the same situation that is being described. In order to be empathic, professionals must be in tune with themselves, know their personal boundaries, and be willing to share their experiences. Boundaries are personal "comfort zones" that define the components of self: body image, personal identity, role performance, self-concept, and self-ideal. Health care professionals must be secure in their personal boundaries in order to develop professional boundaries. The professional can be empathic without the worry of being manipulated. Manipulation results from need. The empathic response of the health care professional will present itself as meeting the needs of the individual, therefore, there is less need for the individual to resort to manipulation.

Like so many other skills, the development of empathy is a process. One is not born empathetic. On the contrary, children can be egocentric and lack the cognitive development needed to understand someone else's point of view. Empathy evolves over time, and professional empathy needs to be cultivated and nurtured. Hammond, Hepworth and Smith (1977) regarded the empathetic process as the creation of the world as we perceive it, rather than our response to it. They see the process moving in a developmental sequence:

- The experience of a biological state whereby persons experience their own bodily actions
- A state where feelings become more differentiated and specific
- Increased awareness of the person's own bodily responses and feelings
- The ability to detect other's needs, feelings, and moods

Empathetic professionals are aware of the uniqueness of clients' feelings. They really care about their client's needs and they create open and effective [affective] communication (Leddy & Pepper, 1993).

Affective communication is a process by which individuals express their feelings. It is a major ingredient in the formation of self-concept, as children form opinions about themselves through affective communication. Empathy is the central focus in affective communication, since empathy is the ability to see the world through the eyes of another —both the joys and the sorrows. Empathy has two components: understanding and response. For the first, professionals must develop the ability to be sensitive to the needs and feelings of clients. To do so requires the ability to read verbal, paralinguistic, and nonverbal cues. For the second, professionals need to be able to respond in a manner that is meaningful and rewarding to the client (*Comptons*, 1996). The latter requires the appropriate intervention skills that develop through education and experience.

Both empathy and affective communication require the ability to listen actively, which means to be attentive to the client's verbal and nonverbal communication.

Active listening can be facilitated by using techniques that can be identified by the acronym SOLER (Townsend, 1996):

S — Sit directly in front of the client giving the message that you are interested in what he or she has to say.

O — Observe an open posture with arms and legs uncrossed. This implies that you are open to what the client has to say. Crossed arms and legs signify "closed" posture and a defensive status. You cannot be empathetic if you are defensive.

L — Lean forward, conveying a sense that you are interested. Make a sincere effort to be attentive.

E — Establish eye contact to convey a willingness to listen to what the client has to say. The absence of eye contact signifies disinterest and even a lack of trust. Trust is a foundation of empathy. (But remember not to stare. That creates discomfort.)

R — Relax to demonstrate your comfort with the client. You cannot be an empathetic listener if you are uncomfortable.

Since empathy also has a cognitive component, individuals can learn to model the behaviors. Health care students in clinical practicums have many opportunities to learn how to be empathic. They should take time to know their clients and actively listen to their stories to better understand client feelings, thoughts, and behaviors. Effective communication skills should be used: lean forward in an interested manner, use eye contact, ask open-ended questions, use a warm/caring tone of voice, be nonjudgmental and respectful. These skills both arise from empathy and demonstrate it. A very effective way to learn empathy is to "walk a mile in the client's shoes." How would you think, feel, and behave if you were a 25-year-old athlete who became completely paralyzed after diving into a shallow pond while intoxicated?

Unfortunately, in some situations the student is told not to be empathic: "If you care too much, you will not be effective." Senior clinicians and teachers need to take the time to embrace situations that allow students to explore their feelings and discuss them openly. What is needed are learning opportunities that will allow them to define their boundaries. If the student is young or inexperienced, role modeling by the senior clinician or teacher can help define their personal boundaries and their professional boundaries.

Clinical experience can be augmented with structured exercises that help individuals recognize situations in which empathy occurs (or could have occurred). These reflective exercises can be completed in a log or journal and submitted to the instructor for feedback. They can also be used in small group discussions to allow students to hear each others' perspective on empathic interventions.

One can learn empathy through service learning. The interest in community and voluntary service grows stronger every day, and the combination of service and learning is intense. Students engage in activities that they and society view as important. These activities necessitate reaching beyond the current range of previous knowledge or experience, and require that the person become an active participant, not a passive spectator (Honnet & Poulsen, 1989). Service learning allows individuals the opportunities to develop empathy by encouraging them to work with varied populations with diverse needs and voices. Students learn to develop sensitivity to barriers such as race, religion, disabilities, lack of transportation, family and other responsibilities, and the uncertainty about one's ability to make a contribution (Honnet & Poulsen, 1989).

Art (both visual and literary) and empathy are viewed as complementary worlds. Peloquin (1996) noted themes connected to empathy: an expression of being there, transforming of the soul, a recognition of likeness and uniqueness, a connection with another's feelings, and the enrichment that comes from these actions. She goes on to note that art elicits three responses that resemble the actions of empathy: response, emotion, and connection.

The empathy response is similar to that found in art. There is an exchange that shapes the understanding of another's reality. Empathy requires an active grasp of the situation and feelings of another. Like art, there is an exchange that moves back and forth from feeling to thought. When a person is empathetic, the action is deep and personally responsive.

Empathy, like art, evokes emotionality. There is a demand for a sensitivity that stops, attends, and grasps someone else's feelings. That heightened sense of the other's emotions may be the transformation of the soul. The fundamental aim of both empathy and art is to make the feeling of brotherhood more customary.

Both empathy and art share connection. Empathy requires a sharing that is personal and nonpredjudiced. Empathetic connections, like those in art, deepen one's sense of reality through compassion.

Health care professionals value empathy as an attitude that affirms human dignity, and concepts from the behavioral sciences suggest that artistic experiences develop empathy. Empathy requires a growing from within the self, a growing that requires the pursuit of experiences that awaken a sense of fellowship. Art philosophers and artists state that the awakening can occur through art (Peloquin, 1996).

Smyth (1996) also promotes artistic expression as a

contributor to the development of empathy. She claims that aesthetic experiences can: allow professionals to gain insight into another person's perspective, allow us to go outside our natural frame of reference, aid us in understanding the needs of clients from other cultures, promote spontaneity and optimism, assist us in dealing with uncertainty and indeterminacy, evoke a sense of unity, and enhance empathy (Smyth, 1996). Think about your favorite book or movie. What made it your favorite? Chances are it was your ability to identify with the hero and understand his or her thoughts, feelings, and actions —even if you didn't agree with them. That's empathy.

Demonstrating Empathy

Charlie (client): *I just don't know what to do. I have so much anger and disappointment in my life that it is difficult to put it in words. My wife told me she's leaving me for another man. I suppose my kids will want to go with her. I know the company I work for is going to close, so I won't have a job in the next few weeks. My world doesn't exist anymore.*

How would you respond to Charlie if he were your friend? How would you respond if he were your client? Are your two responses different?

The ability to respond empathically to others is a learned response. Active listening necessitates extracting the essential themes of the communication and deciding how to identify, prioritize, and respond in a meaningful way. The professional listening to Charlie needs to identify the essential themes that Charlie is experiencing (loss, hopelessness, helplessness, and despair). The professional would then prioritize the themes and respond in a therapeutic manner.

The response of the listener makes a difference. The lay person may say "Gee, that's too bad," leaving the person trapped in a negative experience with little or no outlet for further expression. On the other hand, if the professional responds "It must be difficult to have so many changes," the individual may feel encouraged to continue to discuss his feelings and thoughts because he has felt understood and felt a sense of connection.

I remember a moment in the second grade playing bingo. I didn't win any of the games. My friend, Susan, realized that I felt sad. She looked at me, and without saying a word handed me one of her prizes (I still have it 35 years later!). That is empathy in a child, giving something that is concrete (a prize) to another person. This "gift" of empathy changes as individuals mature. They are less concrete, as empathy on the adult level is abstract and intuitive.

Levels of Development

Novice

Beginning novices are given situations in terms of objective attributes, such as measurements and deadlines. Rules must be followed. Unfortunately, rules cannot convey all professional behaviors, especially one like empathy. Empathy must develop and mature throughout the developmental process. The beginner has only personal experience with empathy, and this experience is the foundation for its professional development. Advanced beginners have coped with real situations enough to learn the aspects of empathy, aspects that can be learned only through experience.

Novices are beginning to learn active listening skills, skills that are critical to the ability to consider the ideas and opinions of others. Empathetic contacts may be occasionally lost during the novices' attempts to clarify what the client is trying to say. Empathy can also become impaired when novices become self-conscious as they struggle to learn their skill and other professional behaviors. However, through experience, careful mentoring, and clinical group discussions, empathy increases as the novice matures in the professional development process.

Apprentice

Competence develops when clinicians see their actions in terms of long-term goals. Plans are based on considerable conscious, abstract, and analytical contemplation of the problem. Apprentices are developing a feeling of mastery and the ability to manage many clinical contingencies. This allows them the ability to be increasingly more empathetic. Competence can be enhanced by planning and coordinating care for more complex clients, enabling the clinician to move toward proficiency.

The more experienced clinician is the one who most frequently notes deterioration or client problems prior to explicit changes. This is due in part to more advanced assessment skills, however, it is also due to increasing empathic ability enabled by the professional's ability to connect with the client. The apprentice is sensitive and responds to the feelings and behaviors of others.

Expert

Due to enormous experiential backgrounds, experts have an intuitive grasp of situations and the ability to zone in on problems without wasting time. However, expertise is not always descriptive because the expert operates from a deep understanding of total situations. They are very effective in detecting early changes and making recommendations due to their ability to perceive the needs of others.

Professionals should render assistance to all individuals without bias or prejudice at all levels of professional development. Yet it is the expert who has the greater strength to provide this assistance to more than just clients. The expert has the empathic ability to fully understand the feelings of peers and colleagues, and uses this ability to respond to their behaviors and to consider their opinions. Proficient professionals share that expertise with others, and they are motivated to develop and nurture young professionals.

Barriers to the Development of Empathy

Even the most proficient professionals have moments when they are not able to be empathetic. Personal problems, lack of sleep, stress, time constraints, and workload can all create barriers to empathy. When significantly stressed, people, including professionals, lose some of their ability to deflect stimuli, increasing their focus on themselves and endangering their ability to be empathetic. Some professionals find it difficult to be empathetic with specific clients, such as persons who commit crimes like murder and child sexual assault; others find it difficult to empathize with persons who react differently from the expected norm.

Health care professionals must make themselves aware of these barriers and they must be able to recognize when they or other professionals are facing them. Discussions with peers, teachers, and supervisors assist in creating this awareness. Once aware of the situation, professionals can respond either by becoming more empathetic, or removing themselves from the relationship. The latter, which may be necessary when dealing with clients whose values significantly clash with yours, must be dealt with in a manner that is still nonjudgmental and respectful. The professional is also responsible for seeing that another professional be consulted to provide the empathetic relationship with that client.

Case Stories/Anecdotal Vignettes

Lack of Empathy and Effects

Clarice, 22, has been drug-dependent for 10 years. She is 7 months pregnant and is having her first prenatal visit and ultrasound. The technician determines the presence of a cranial malformation and informs Clarice of his findings. Clarice turns to him and starts to cry, asking "How could something like this happen?" The technician looks at Clarice and responds, "You should have thought of that before you got pregnant. What did you think would happen if you continued to abuse drugs and got pregnant?"

Unfortunately, the technician's value system impaired his ability to be empathic. The client becomes overwhelmed by anxiety, guilt, and loss, leaving her with the need to seek relief. Substance-abusing individuals are unlikely to use effective coping mechanisms, and therefore Clarice is likely to seek comfort in her drug of choice.

Presence of Empathy and Effects

Michael is celebrating his 21st birthday confined to a rehabilitation facility for treatment of quadriplegia after a diving accident. He is angered and depressed by his condition and sees no foreseeable future for himself and his fianceé. Michael's therapist understands his dilemma. He plans a quiet birthday party for just Michael and his fianceé and makes arrangements for the fianceé to present Michael with a motorized wheelchair that he can control through head movements. The therapist wheels the fianceé in on the wheelchair and she leans over, kisses Michael and says, "I'll always love you." Michael smiles for the first time in weeks.

Empathy has many guises, and actions speak louder than words. The professional recognized Michael's feelings and needs and responded to them with actions that demonstrated that he really cared for his client. The therapist also utilized the empathy of a loved one, Michael's fianceé, which is a powerful force that should never be overlooked. Michael, in turn, realized that someone was there for him, someone who understood how he was feeling. That and the knowledge that he still had a future to look forward to are critical components in his struggle to reach his optimal level of health.

Sometimes, it's the little things that we do that mean the most to clients. These gestures work because they evolve from empathy.

References

Abraham, K., Kuehl, R., & Christopherson, U. (1983). *Child Study Journal, 13(3),* 175-185.

Baillie, L. (1996). A phenomenological study of the nature of empathy. *Journal of Advanced Nursing, 24,* 1300-1308.

Barrett-Lennard, G. T. (1981). The empathy cycle: Refinement of a nuclear concept. *Journal of Counseling Psychology, 28(9),* 91-100.

Brent, D. (1985). Psychiatric assessment of the school aged child. *Psychiatric Annuals, 75(1),* 30-33.

Brunt, J. H. (1985). An exploration of the relationship between nurses' empathy and technology. *Nursing Administration Quarterly, 9(45),* 69-78.

Comptons Living Encyclopedia. Comptons Learning Co., 1996. (On line.) America Online (7 June 1996).

Christiansen, C. (1977). Measuring empathy in occupational therapy students. *The American Journal of Occupational Therapy, 31(1),* 19-22.

Davis, M. (1983). Measuring individual differences in empathy: Evidence for a multidimensional approach. *Journal of Personality and Social Psychology, 44(1),* 113-186.

Davis, M., Luce, C., & Kraus, S. (1994). The heritability of characteristics associated with dispositional empathy. *Journal of Personality, 62(3),* 369-392.

Dymond, R. (1949). A scale for the measurement of empathic ability. *Journal of Consulting Psychologist, 12,* 127-133.

Emde, R. (1985). An adaptive view of infant emotions: Functions for self and knowing. *Social Science Information, 24(2),* 337-341.

Fabes, R., Eisenberg, N., Karborn, M., Troyer, D., & Switzer, G. (1994). The relationship of children's emotion regulation to their vicarious emotional responses and comforting behaviors. *Child Development, 65(6),* 1678-1694.

Forsyth, G. (1980). Analysis of the concept of empathy: Illustration of one approach. *Advances in Nursing Science, 3(1),* 33-42.

Freeman, E. (1984). The development of empathy in young children: In search of a definition. *Child Study Journal, 13(4),* 235-245.

Gagan, J. (1983). Methodological notes on empathy. *Advances in Nursing Science, 16(1),* 65-72.

Gibbs, J. & Woll, S. (1985). Mechanisms used by young children in the making of empathic judgments. *Journal of Personality, 53,(4),* 575-585.

Gladstein, G. (1983). Understanding empathy: Integrating counseling, developmental, and social psychology perspectives. *Journal of Counseling Psychology, 30,* 407-482.

Gnepp, J., Klayman, J. & Trabasso, T. (1982). A hierarchy of information sources for inferring emotional reactions. *Journal of Experimental Child Psychology, 20(3),* 280-284.

Goldstein, A. & Michaels, G. (1985). *Empathy development, training, and consequences.* Hillsdale, NJ: Lawrence Erlbaum Associates, Publishers.

Grief, E. and Hogan, R. (1973). The theory and measurement of empathy. *Journal of Counseling Psychologist, 20(3),* 280-284.

Hammond, D. C, Hepworth, D. H., and Smith, V. G. (1977). *Improving therapeutic communication.* San Francisco, CA: Jossey-Bass.

Hogan, R. (1969). Development of an empathy scale. *Journal of Consulting and Clinical Psychology, 33(3),* 307-316.

Hogan, R. (1975). Empathy: A conceptual and psychometric analysis. *The Counseling Psychologist, 5(2),* 14-18.

Honnet, E., & Poulsen, S. (1989). *Principles of good practice for combining service and learning.* Racine, WI: The Johnson Foundation, Inc.

Jordan, J. (1983). *Empathy and the mother-daughter relationship.* Work in Progress No. 82-02. Wellesley, MA: The Stone Center for Developmental Services and Studies.

LaMonica, E. (1979). Empathy in nursing practice. *Issues In Mental Health Nursing, 2(1),* 1-13.

Leddy, S. & Pepper, J. (1993). *Conceptual basis of professional nursing,* 3rd Edition. Philadelphia, PA: JB Lippincott Co.

Lipps, T. (1909). *Leitfaden der psychologie.* Leipzig, Germany: Englemann.

Morgan, S. (1983). Development of emotionally disturbed children. *Journal of Humanistic Education and Development, 22(2),* 70-79.

O'Toole, M. (1997). *Miller-Keane encyclopedia & dictionary of medicine, nursing, and alied health,* 6th Edition. Philadelphia, PA: W. B. Saunders Co.

Peloquin, S. (1996). Art: An occupation with promise for developing empathy. *The American Journal of Occupational Therapy, 50(8),* 655-661.

Scavo, R., & Buchanan, B. (1989). Group therapy for male adolescent sex offenders: A model for residential treatment. *Residential Treatment for Children and Youth, 7(2),* 59-74.

Schulman, L. (1984). The prevention of antisocial behavior through moral motivation training: or Why isn't there more street crime? *Prevention in Human Services, 1(1),* 255-275.

Smith, H. C. (1973). *Sensitivity training: The scientific understanding of individuals.* New York, NY: McGraw-Hill Book Company.

Smyth, T. (1996). Reinstating the person in the professional: Reflections on empathy and aesthetic experience. *Journal of Advanced Nursing, 24,* 932-937.

Surrey, J. (1985). *Self-in-relationship: A theory of women's development.* Work in Progress No. 13. Wellesley, MA: The Stone Center for Developmental Services and Studies.

Townsend, M. (1996). *Psychiatric mental health nursing: Concepts of care,* 2nd Edition. Philadelphia, PA: FA Davis.

Traux, C. (1961). A scale for the measurement of accurate empathy. *Psychiatric Institute Bulletin, 1,* 12-21.

Wheeler, K. (1988). A nursing science approach to understanding empathy. *Archives of Psychiatric Nursing, 2(2),* 95-100.

Wise, B. & Page, M. (1980). Empathy levels of occupational therapy students. *The American Journal of Occupational Therapy, 34(10),* 676-679.

World Book Encyclopedia (1968). Chicago, IL: Thorndike-Barnhart Dictionary Series.

Ungerer, J., Dolby, R., Waters, B., Barnette, B., et. al. (1990). The early development of empathy: Self-regulation and individual differences in the first year. *Motivation-and-Emotion, 14(2),* 93-106.

Zahn-Waxler, C., & Radke-Yarrow, M. (1990). The origins of empathic concern. *Motivation-and-Emotion, 14(2),* 107-130.

Exercises to Develop Empathy

The following exercises may be done in individual journal format, in small group discussion, or a combination of the two.

These case studies are not meant to confuse you. These scenarios are as vague as they would be in real clinical situations. They are meant to help you think and relate in an empathetic manner.

1. You're late for your next appointment. As you charge down the hall, you pass a young fireman sitting in a wheel-chair, crying as he stares at his fully bandaged hands. The nearby bedside table holds a photo of the man and a young woman holding a little boy. The table is covered with milk spilled from a fallen glass. The man looks up at you and says, "I thought I was doing the right thing. Was I?"
   A. What do you perceive from this situation?
   B. What could the man be talking about? What could he be feeling? How would you find out the answer to these questions?
   C. How would you handle this situation? Now, consider your response; is it empathetic? If so, why is it? If not, why not?
   D. How did you feel abut this situation?

2. You are working with an elderly woman who is dying. She has been ill for a long time and was a victim of the Holocaust. You sit with her and hold her hand. She states, "Go. Go to someone who needs you. I am an old woman who is very used to dying. I've seen much of it and now it is my time to be with God. Go, I will be fine."
   A. What do you perceive from this situation?
   B. What could the woman be talking about? What could she be feeling? How would you find out the answer to these questions?
   C. How would you handle this situation? Now, consider your response; is it empathetic? If so, why is it? If not, why not?
   D. How did you feel about this situation?

3. Use your artistic expression. Paint, draw, write, tell, or act out a story — from someone else's point of view. Think, feel, and act as if you are one of the following persons:
   A. A 4-year-old who is hospitalized for the first time and who is all alone.
   B. A developmentally-delayed adult who is having a full body CAT scan and cannot understand directions.
   C. A 75-year-old woman whose husband of more than 50 years has just died.
   D. A 13-year-old whose leg was amputated in an auto accident.
   E. A 50-year-old woman experiencing menopause.
   F. A 50-year-old male experiencing a mid-life crisis.
   G. Come up with your own idea or fictionalize the story of a client that you worked with.

4. Participate in a support group that has open admission. Check the blue pages in your phone book or ask for information at your school's counseling center. Discuss empathetic encounters with the group leader.

5. Participate in service learning. If your school does not have a program, encourage them to start one.

Additional Resources

1. Search the word "empathy" on the Internet to see how many different aspects you can learn.
2. Davis, M. (1996). *Empathy: A social psychological approach.* New York, NY: Harper Collins Publishers.

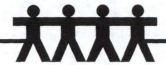

Chapter Eight

Cooperation

Marlene J. Morgan, MOT, OTR/L

To cooperate is to work with one or more persons (Mish, 1986). A group that is cooperating works toward a common goal or for a common purpose. As a professional in health care, you most often will experience cooperation in the workplace as an important component of a larger construct — teamwork. This chapter will improve your understanding of cooperation, teams, and teamwork by addressing the following questions:

What skills do you need to develop before entering into a cooperative relationship?

How is a team different from a group?

What makes an effective team?

How do teams form?

What will your role on a team be?

Why is there so much attention paid today to teams in health care and business?

Are you ready to be a cooperative team member?

How will your understanding of and involvement in teams change throughout your career?

Foundations of Cooperation

Cooperation is a complex concept. Cooperation is demonstrated by someone who works effectively with other individuals, shows consideration for the needs of the group, and develops group cohesiveness by facilitating the knowledge and awareness of others (Kasar, Clark, Watson & Pfister, 1996). Prior to entering into a rela-tionship requiring cooperation, an individual must establish and demonstrate a series of professional behaviors. Dependability, professional presentation, initiative, empathy, clinical reasoning, and verbal communication (these are professional behaviors discussed in other chapters) are skills foundational to cooperation. Dependability is key to demonstrating consideration for the needs of a group. Effective professional presentation is critical to group acceptance and the ability of an individual to facilitate the knowledge and awareness of others. Initiative relates to the ability of an individual to promote group knowledge and problem-solving. Empathy allows a person to show consideration for both individual and group thoughts and actions. Sound clinical reasoning ensures that an individual will bring to the cooperative relationship ideas and solutions to move the goal of the group forward. Effective verbal communication allows for clear and concise interactions among group members. Attention to the development of each of these characteristics will provide you with a firm foundation of knowledge and interpersonal skills on which to build cooperative relationships.

Cooperation In Teams and Groups

Teamwork and cooperation are easy to recognize and to talk about, but hard to make happen. Bringing people together in a group does not guarantee that they will cooperate and form or work as a team. There are three clear distinctions between a group and a team. One key way that a team is different from a group is that the members of a team most often have well-defined positions. An interdisciplinary heath care team may consist of a nurse, doctor, PT, OT, social worker, dietician, speech pathologist, audiologist, and medical ethics consultant. Each individual member holds a distinct position in the organization and brings to the team a unique body of professional knowledge and a set of technical skills. One member may be a leader in his department while another may be a junior member or a part-time employee. On the team, each is representing not only himself but also the expertise of his field to move the team forward toward accomplishing its goal. As a group forms a team, each member finds and forms roles for himself in the structure of the team. His role on the team may not be the one that he plays in the organization at large. For example, a supervisor in the OT department may not assume a leadership role on the team, but will support the leadership of a staff nurse who works for the organization part-time. As you approach team membership be aware that position in an organization does not automatically translate to position on a team. A second distinguishing characteristic is the fact that team members are drawn together toward a common goal or for a common purpose. Teams that share common goals and objectives based on core beliefs and values make some of the most effective decisions and solve the most complex problems. Organizations call on teams to cooperate and solve a series of problems over time. This is the third way that a team can be distinguished from a group. Now take a look at some effective teams demonstrating cooperation in action.

An interdisciplinary team working in home care meets to discuss Mr. Misner. Mr. Misner is living at home and wants to remain there but is having a difficult time. A recent fall has sent him to the hospital with a broken hip. As hospital discharge approaches, the decision is made to send him home rather than to the rehabilitation hospital. A home care nurse, PT, OT, and social worker meet to develop a plan designed to provide Mr. Misner with adaptive equipment to use at home during his recovery, encourage him to improve his ability to walk as his hip heals, provide for meals on wheels, enlist a home health aid to assist with housework temporarily, and monitor him for compliance with a new medication. The social worker takes the lead in the discussion. This team has formed around the common goal of providing Mr. Misner

with optimum conditions to allow for his independence at home. Each team member values independence and a patient's right to live where he chooses provided that health and safety are not compromised. The successful implementation of their cooperative plan will achieve that goal.

In an acute care hospital, the members of a heart transplant team meet to design an orientation process for nurses new to the unit. Through the reading materials they choose, the lectures that they design, and the technical checkouts that they recommend, the members of this team are demonstrating their cooperation, commitment, and value to the goals of providing effective, efficient, and high quality patient care on the transplant unit. The successful implementation of their plan will contribute to these goals.

Upstairs in the administrative offices the management committee, consisting of the hospital administrator and the directors of nursing, clinical nutrition, and medicine, meet to review proposals submitted by rival food service companies to provide healthy meals for the institution. Each is interested in the important role that good nutrition plays in the recovery process and values the role that food plays in restoring health. At the same time they are aware of the high cost of a hospital stay and committed to keeping expenses under control. At the conclusion of the meeting this team chooses the vendor that offers the best combination of high quality meals and low cost. The execution of the completed contract with the selected vendor will help them meet their goals.

Imagine that you were present at these meetings taking notes and observing. You would see that each team works because it demonstrates the three key components of successful teams: commitment, collaboration, and communication.

Commitment is a concept that comes to life in the values and beliefs that a team has toward its goals. Commitment is demonstrated by team members who arrive at a meeting on time, come prepared, voice their concerns and opinions, are willing to work to achieve and implement the best solution to a problem, and are willing to try again in the face of failure.

Collaboration occurs on a team when members "put their heads together" to identify innovative solutions to problems and brainstorm the best course of action. By listening closely you can hear collaboration illustrated in the language that team members use. When you hear phrases like "let's figure how we can...", "let's decide on a plan for...", "let's talk about...", you are witnessing collaboration in action. Team talk replaces "I" think with "we" think (Navarra, Lipkowitz, & Navarra, 1990). Collaborative effort means that all participants share in success and failure. When the team does well members pat each other on the back, and when the team experiences failure members reflect on the past and make plans to move forward.

Communication is a key component of team success. Skillful team members foster the exchange and processing of ideas, build relationships, manage conflict, and achieve goals by engaging in open communication. Navarra, Lipkowitz, and Navarra (1990) have identified a system for studying communication patterns on a team. Using this system as a guide, your analysis of the communication patterns on a successful team would reveal members who:

• Acknowledge Expertise: Each professional is valued for the knowledge base, insight, and technical skill he brings to team discussions and the decision-making process.

• Observe Subtle Cues: The effective team member not only listens but looks for cues or messages from others that add meaning to what is being said. Cues may be hidden in body language or voice quality or tone.

• Dig Beneath the Surface: Teams are frequently formed to deal with complex problems. Communication on the team encourages members to behave as detectives seeking as much information from as many sources as possible. Questions and follow-up questions are most often used to "dig."

• Show Acceptance: Teams work because of the variety of personalities and opinions present. Accepting that someone has the right to an opinion does not imply agreement, but an openness to listening to other views in a nonjudgmental way.

• Know When To Be Quiet: At times the best contribution a team member can make to a discussion is to be quiet.

• Clarify Meaning: As discussions progress on a team, it is important for a group to stop periodically and restate the key points. This process allows discussions to move forward free of misunderstandings.

• Express Healthy Skepticism: Effective team members speak up to make their voices heard when they do not agree with discussion points or the proposed plan. Healthy skepticism is never an attack on the team or an individual, rather it is a request to view an issue from a different perspective.

• Assess Progress: Teams are goal-oriented and value-driven. Assessing progress is required to insure that discussions, decisions, and actions are moving the team in the right direction.

Remember Mr. Misner who you met earlier in the chapter? His team has invited you to listen in on their meeting. As you read the dialog, listen for evidence of cooperation and effective communication.

Scene: Social work office at University Hospital. A team consisting of a social worker, nurse, OT, and PT are meeting to discuss progress on Mr. Misner's case.

Social Worker: "We have only three more home care visits approved for Mr. Misner. I think that he will be ready for discharge by then."

OT: "When I was there on Tuesday he and his wife asked if he would be able to walk without the walker. He feels that he does not need it anymore. I said that I would bring it up here at the meeting and seek the advice of PT."

PT: "Did he say why he does not want to use the walker?"

OT: "Yes, he says it is clumsy."

PT: "Is he having difficulty using it in the house?"

OT: "No, not in the house - outside."

(The nurse is looking intently at the occupational therapist but allows her to continue.)

Nurse: "I am not sure that taking away the walker is a good idea. Mr. Misner gets dizzy at times from the medication and without the walker he grabs onto the furniture for support. That is not safe. His wife told me that he is ashamed to be seen with the walker because it makes him feel disabled."

PT: "Oh I see that is the reason. I will talk to him today and re-evaluate him. Maybe a cane would be appropriate for him now."

Careful examination of this dialog illustrates for you good examples of team cooperation and communication.

Development of Cooperative Teams

Teams form by following a developmental process. Just as you moved through rolling, sitting, and standing on your way to walking, the team passes through stages. Tuckman (1965) classified team development into four phases: forming, storming, norming, and performing. Let us examine each stage to identify the characteristics and dynamics of the developing team. Forming is the first phase of team development. At this time the members are social and tentative with each other. They try to get to know each other. Many of the members may have questions about the purpose of the group. In time and through interaction, the team moves into the storming phase. The storming phase is often characterized by conflict as members fight for power and status in the group. During this time ideas and procedures develop. When the storm begins to weaken, the team moves into the norming phase. The team develops "norms" or accepted ways of behaving, becomes cohesive, and really begins to work. Members are willing to put aside individual differences for the sake of the team moving forward. The final phase of development is performing. In this last and most advanced phase the team is able to do its best work. Teams experience increased success during this phase and members report satisfaction and pride.

Your experiences as a team member will be directly related to the phase of development that characterizes the team. Knowledge of this process will enable you to identify the current phase of each team that you find yourself a part of, and suggest strategies that you can use to help the team grow.

Roles of Members

As a professional facing the prospect of working on a team you cannot help but ask and maybe be concerned about the role that you will play. Review of the issues addressed earlier in the chapter makes it easy to construct an image of a team as being flexible and dynamic. Membership on a team is dynamic and flexible too. You do not become a team member to play only one role. Analysis of teams in action allows us to identify and describe several roles you may be asked to play (Navarra, Lipkowitz, & Navarra, 1990).

- Information Seeker: Looks for facts and clarification.
- Opinion Seeker: Exposes the values that underlie team decisions.
- Information giver: Gives facts based on knowledge and experience.
- Opinion Giver: Expresses beliefs and values and suggests them to the group.
- Elaborator: Expands, clarifies, and anticipates the outcomes of decisions.
- Conductor: Combines, coordinates and suggests the relationship among ideas.
- Orienter: Surveys the process, raises questions, and provides direction.
- Evaluator: Compares the group process to performance.

- Recorder: Documents team process to allow the group to see tangible results.

Encouraging role change among members keeps a team energized and active. While you may first feel comfortable with only a few roles, be prepared to expand your roles as your experience in teamwork grows.

Revisit the team meeting dialog for Mr. Misner to see if you are able to identify the role(s) being played by the nurse, social worker, PT, and OT.

Role of Teams in Business and Health Care Today

A shift in thinking is occurring today in business, health care, and education. This shift is happening in response to pressures to contain cost, provide quality service and cater to the needs of customers. Pressure may come from sources as diverse as insurance payers or parents of special needs children. Problems facing business, health care, and education are complex and consumer demands are high. In the past there was very little need for departments to work together, and communication and interaction between professionals was rare. The new world of work is placing a strong emphasis on using cooperative strategies such as teams to solve problems and improve communication. While each profession has an area of expertise and skills, none is able to face complex problems alone. None has all of the information skills and technology to form the best solution. Cooperation and teamwork is the way more and more work will be accomplished. Organizations are beginning to realize that clearly defined jobs are an inhibitor to getting work done. The focus is moving from the more traditional model of "doing a job" or "playing a role" to a broader view of the work that needs to be done and problems that need to be solved (Muller-Smith, 1995). Employers are becoming increasingly sensitive to the fact that they must make maximum use of their best asset to remain competitive (Jacobs, 1995). The best asset of a company, school, or health care system is the people. Employee teams in many organizations today are described as the "motivational glue" that keeps the company focused and together (McKee, 1993). Teamwork and cooperation will play vital roles in our search to successfully compete in all industries both within the United States and abroad (Wojslaw, 1993). The interest in using teams to solve problems and provide services today is a concept that is both popular and promising.

Developing Skills

Real teamwork and cooperation do not come naturally to most people, they need to be learned and developed. Teamwork and cooperation are key to being a successful adult in all areas of life. You cannot run a business, be an employee, or make a marriage work without being team-oriented. If you reflect on your past you will discover a wide range of experiences to build on to develop teamwork skills. You may first have learned to cooperate and be a team member at home. Many families plan vacations, religious celebrations, and projects that provide members with the opportunity to experience and participate in the communication, cooperation, sharing and dedication characteristic of teamwork. At school your involvement in group projects and cooperative learning experiences provided you with the opportunity to work on a team. Assessing group needs, helping each other gather information, preparing joint presentations, and receiving a group grade were valuable lessons in teamwork. You may also have learned how to deal with a group member who did not do his share of the work! Part-time work and volunteer experience presented you with opportunities to develop skills in both cooperation and competition. Competition and teamwork develop hand in hand and enhance each other. While becoming a professional representative to an interdisciplinary team may indeed be a new experience, you have a foundation of past experience to build on and develop.

Teamwork and Career Development

As you reflect on and plan your professional career path, your ability to contribute to the successful functioning of teams will become an important factor. Your progression from novice to apprentice to advanced practitioner will provide unique challenges to your development of teamwork skills.

A novice or entry level professional is concerned with developing a career path for himself. At this stage you look for opportunities that allow you to reach your individual career goals. Novices develop the cooperation skills required for successful team participation as they begin to realize that everyone, with a little help from others, accomplishes and learns more than they could working alone.

At the apprentice stage of development the professional many times faces a dilemma. Being a good team member at this stage frequently takes much thought and work because you may find yourself competing with your peers for time off, resources, and promotions. At this stage it is important to remember that good cooperation and teamwork are vital to the smooth operation of the organization. You can contribute to the organization by promoting teamwork among others at your level. The apprentice promotes teamwork by:

- Communicating openly
- Giving credit where it is due
- Recognizing the need to do more than his share
- Sharing ideas and opportunities
- Sharing the risk as well as the credit for untried solutions

Being an active and involved team member at this stage can lead to the apprentice fulfilling his or her own need for success. Effective teams of apprentices are frequently recognized by administration and empowered to make decisions.

The expert professional is often charged with the responsibility for encouraging cooperation and facilitating teams. In the workplace of today and in the future, fostering teamwork will be important because there will be fewer managers and decisions will be pushed further down into the organization. As an expert you will be viewed as a leader and charged with the responsibility of fostering an atmosphere that will allow for staff and teams to grow and develop. We can check the effectiveness of an expert by comparing his performance to the following list:

- Encourages information sharing
- Provides feedback
- Is flexible and encourages flexibility
- Exhibits trust
- Is available to team members
- Contributes to the organization by doing his own job
- Learns from his mistakes
- Has a sense of humor and can have fun
- Helps staff see the big picture
- Values competence, background, and experience
- Approaches issues and conflicts with a positive mind set
  (Adapted from Muller-Smith, 1995)

The leader of the future who follows this advice will find himself giving up control, exchanging the role of boss for that of a facilitator, and depending on the expertise of the staff. If you are successful in engendering enthusiasm in your staff as the result of being part of a team reaching for a common goal, you will be surprised at how much can be done!

A demonstrated record of cooperating and team success can impact your career path in significant ways. Your ability to collaborate with and manage people will be a critical quality addressed in job performance for promotion and merit. Having a reputation as a team player will open avenues to you for inclusion in committees and professional organizations. Presentations at conferences and election to offices are career enhancers. Dialog with successful leaders in your profession about their career paths will highlight many examples of cooperation and teamwork.

Conclusion

Return to the questions that were posed at the beginning of the chapter. Are you now able to answer one or more of them?

What skills do you need to develop before entering into a cooperative relationship?

How is a team different from a group?

What makes an effective team?

How do teams form?

What will your role on a team be?

Why is there so much attention paid today to teams in health care and business?

Are you ready to be a cooperative team member?

How will your understanding of and involvement on teams change throughout your career?

You are challenged to use these questions as a guide for you to develop skills in cooperation and teamwork. The answers to the questions will change as you grow, and new pressures and challenges for professionals emerge.

References

Jacobs, R. (1995, February). Workers strive for more voice in decision-making. *Michigan Nurse,* 12-13.

Kasar, J., Clark, E. N., Watson, D., & Pfister, S. (1996). *Professional Development Assessment.* Unpublished form.

McKee, B. (1993, July). Turn your workers into a team. *Nation's Business,* 36-38.

Mish, F. (Ed.). (1986). *Webster's ninth new collegiate dictionary.* Springfield, MA: Merriam-Webster.

Muller-Smith, P. (1995). Tomorrow's workplace: No jobs... just work to be done. *Journal of Post Anesthesia Nursing, 10,* 172-174.

Navarra, T., Lipkowitz, M., & Navarra, J. (1990). *Therapeutic communication: A guide to effective interpersonal skills for health care professionals.* Thorofare, NJ: SLACK Incorporated.

Tuckman, B. (1965). Developmental sequence in small groups. *Psychological Bulletin, 63,* 384-399.

Wojslaw, C. F. (1993, Winter). Teamwork and community. *IEEE Technology and Society Magazine,* 23-27.

Exercises to Develop Cooperation

1. Participate in or observe a group. Look for evidence of commitment, collaboration and communication. Reflect on your experience or observation. Was the team effective or not?

2. Interview someone in your field who is considered "successful." Question that person about his or her feelings regarding the importance of cooperation and the role teams have played in his or her career.

3. Participate in a team meeting or discussion and reflect on the roles that you played and the communication patterns that you exhibited. Were you a good team member? Were you cooperative? List areas that you would like to focus on for improved team membership. Write a short action plan for each area.

Additional Resources

There are many excellent resources available to the professional interested in understanding cooperation and teams. The following suggestions address team development and communication. Each gives practical suggestions for developing your skills.

Navarra, T., Lipkowitz, M., & Navarra, J. (1990). *Therapeutic communication: A guide to effective interpersonal skills for health care professionals.* Thorofare, NJ: SLACK Incorporated.

Bridges, W. (1991). *Managing transitions.* New York, NY: Addison-Wesley.

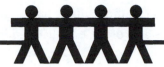

Chapter Nine

Organization

E. Nelson Clark,
MS, OTR/L

"Come on guys, lets get organized!" This was a frequent comment from Moe to Larry and Curley in the classic comedies of the *Three Stooges* (Maurer, 1984). The remark was usually made after a disastrous, but amusing, attempt at getting started.

Definition

Organize: to begin, start, initiate, create, and establish a category, arrangement, array, and give order to an activity, assignment, undertaking, or a venture (*Webster's* 1981).

immaculate living situation while his roommate Oscar is the opposite and brings confusion and disorder in a comic manner (Simon, 1966).

Laughter at the farcical performances of these comedians appears in the form of comic relief. Although the incidents are happening to the comedian, we vicariously associate some of our own actions at those times when we are not so organized. Most readers would readily agree that it is more humorous to see others in a panic, bumbling their way through a predicament, than it is to see ourselves in the same situation.

Disorganization can be Humorous

Laughter is often directed at the organizationally challenged. The antics of the early screen movies and vaudevillian acts, such as the *Three Stooges* and the *Keystone Cops*, illustrated that the inability to organize often leads to disastrous results. In the case of these comedians, the lack of planning often led to hitting someone across the head with a long piece of lumber or striking significant body parts that inflicted howling pain. The call for immediate and corrective action resulted in individuals running around in circles in a panic and often running back into each other. The disorganized behaviors of comedians are timeless.

Humor is sometimes directed at the individual who attempts to over-organize situations, such as the character Felix in the *Odd Couple*, who attempts to maintain an

The Need for Organization

Recounting the occasional incident of disorganization may add humor and spice to one's conversational reminiscing; however, the inability to organize yourself is not humorous in the performance of indispensable daily living skills and in the essential need of generating income in one's employment. Laughter is soon turned to concern and sadness when we see disease and trauma affect the skills necessary to feed, dress, or wash yourself, and take care of such basic tasks as cooking, cleaning, and maintaining living quarters.

The inability to organize basic life skills is often the first clue of an acute illness. As benign as the common cold, or as disruptive as the flu, when the illness begins we often find ourselves unable to concentrate, organize simple tasks, or even feed or dress ourselves in order to go to work.

An individual can be mistakenly accused of willful incompetence or simply not caring in the early stages of a disease that results in dysfunction. The individual may not exhibit the skill or productivity that he or she once displayed. They may adapt excuses or avoidances for difficulty in certain tasks or administrative functions. Then, as the disease process unfolds, we begin to understand the reasons for the dysfunctional behaviors. We watch helplessly as a disease process such as Alzheimer's slowly diminishes the highly competent organizational skills of the individual (Smoller, 1997).

No example serves us better in recent times than the case of the former President of the United States, Ronald Reagan. President Reagan was a popular movie actor in his young adulthood. Later he became Governor of California and a respected statesman, and then was elected to the office of United States Presidency in 1980 and 1984. His administrative, communication, and interpersonal skills were of the highest order as he functioned as the world's most powerful leader. So much so, that his negotiation skills were attributed to the dismantling of the Berlin Wall that separated the free world (West Germany) from communist-held (East Germany) countries. However, in Reagan's last presidential years we can now see a withdrawal from the public and an increased intervention of his cabinet members into the governing of the affairs of the country. His wife, Nancy, was also criticized at the time for increased intervention and control of his personal life. We can now gain a historical perspective for the changed behaviors of President Reagan and those closest to him. He was in the early stages of Alzheimer's disease. He now resides under close nursing care in his home and makes rare public appearances. When he does make an appearance, it's usually just a brief hand wave to the camera in order to maintain the dignity of this great man.

In order to understand and perhaps even predict the onset of various illnesses, we should examine the history and skills of an individual's ability to effectively organize. We should also understand the component processes of organization. The first step of this process is an individual's ability to simply function.

The Function of Organization

Organizational skills, by the earlier definition, appear to be in two areas of function: the first is being able to initiate, begin, and create the thought process necessary to establish order.

The inabilities or difficulties encountered in this stage frequently lead to a "procrastination period," which is the delay or stalling that inhibits the initiation of a project for a certain length of time (Burka & Yuen, 1983). Procrastination has many facets to deterring an individual from accomplishment (Sapadin & Maguire, 1996). An individual can be deterred from performing activities as basic as self-care or as sophisticated as writing this chapter for a book on professional behaviors. During the procrastination period, individuals may delay the necessary performance of a task for many reasons. For example, he or she may be frustrated at the current situation of not having enough perceived income. He or she might spend time daydreaming of winning the lottery to the point of being non-functional in their required activity. An older individual who cannot organize the simple daily living task of putting on a shirt or blouse, may procrastinate by telling a story of when he or she was younger and able to work effectively. These delaying behaviors are often symptoms that indicate a change in habits and lifestyle. In order to better understand these procrastinating behaviors, the health care practitioner must examine the individual's organizing skills, assist in recognizing organizational losses, and develop strategies to help regain those skills.

Different from a disease or injury process are the individuals who are able to effectively use and channel the procrastination period into creative endeavors (Porat, 1980). The delay of participation in a task or activity is sometimes referred to as a "mulling period". This mulling period or process occurs in the mind while the individual ponders, weighs, or thinks over what is needed to initiate a productive course of action. We often see this process in coffee shops, break rooms, or around the water cooler, where people are attempting to "get started" in the mornings. Many individuals use a drug such as caffeine or nicotine to aid in the process of waking up or getting started to assist in organizing their first thoughts of the day. Some people use forms of exercise such as jogging, tai chi, stretching, or meditation to increase the flow of mind-enhancing nutrients such as oxygen, blood, and adrenaline. And then there are some who shut off the alarm in the morning and refuse to get out of bed until the last second. This "last second" syndrome provides a panic that stimulates the body to produce adrenaline that pumps through the body's system and gives enough importance to being on time for work, school, or to perform a critical task. A number of professionals from athletes to actors use the stimulation of adrenaline to assist in getting started. The modern term "getting pumped up" for action involves getting the level of the whole system increased to handle additional workloads.

Whatever method one chooses to initiate the first phase of organization will likely develop life-long habits that determine how successful or functional one is in his or her organizing skills. However, the habits that one might build in coping with the early stages of organization may not be sufficient for organizing higher levels of performance required in more challenging roles. For example, if one has acquired a habit of drinking coffee to rely on caffeine to get the mind boosted for simple activities, he or she might find that drinking excess coffee will later impair certain thinking and fine motor skills (Gilbert, 1986). Also, while rolling out of bed at the last moment and not eating breakfast might work for high school, is it a good health habit for college or employment?

Medical Assessment

The inability to get started with symptoms of confusion, memory impairment, fine or gross motor incoordination, or other sensory disturbance, is cause for immediate and complete medical examination. Neurological disturbances often involve separate areas of the brain that are interrelated in a very complicated fashion. The inability to organize may also be accompanied by the loss of meaningful speech or sensory loss to an area of the body.

An individual who has been acutely injured (such as a head trauma), or one who has experienced long-term or severe chemical abuse (such as drugs or alcohol), may see early signs of deterioration in simple organizational skills and neurological functions.

While it is not the intent of this chapter to go into extensive neurological explanations of disease processes, the practicing health care professional should recognize the earliest symptoms of the inability to organize, and consult or refer to a professional who is experienced in the area of neurological functioning. These individuals can assist in timely identification and diagnosis of disorders that are manifested by early signs of disorganization. For example, a thorough cognitive assessment may detect an individual's inability to organize thought into meaningful action.

Organization as Meaningful Order

Meaningful action is the second component of organizing. It is the skill or ability to place thoughts and actions into meaningful order. To be able to arrange, array, and prioritize one's thoughts into actions often determines how successfully one functions. Successful behaviors in this area lead to being able to quickly determine what is needed in a particular situation and being able to pursue a confident course of action. Courses of action can be as varied as dressing yourself for lounging around the house in pajamas, or awakening in the firehouse to an alarm and donning sophisticated firefighting equipment in a matter of seconds.

The ability to quickly arrange thoughts and actions into meaningful order, as viewed in analytical psychiatry, is the ability to "control instinctual drives" (Horner, 1991). Instinctual drives are the behaviors of aggressive and sexual forces that build experiences that comprise organizing principles for mental behaviors. Developmentally speaking, an individual successfully progresses through life by learning or acquiring appropriate experiences. These positive experiences enable one to develop appropriate thought processes, and thus acceptable outward behaviors according to societal norms. Interruption of this process can occur through various illnesses, traumatic injuries, and chemical abuse. Examples of the inability to control impulsive aggressive and sexual drives are evident daily on the front pages of your local newspaper. Normal and appropriate methods to control impulses allow individuals to delay and organize acceptable releases for these instinctual drives.

Capacity for Delay

In order to effectively control instinctual drives, one must have a certain *capacity for delay*. This delay action will allow thoughts to be placed in a meaningful order to enable an individual to pursue a functional action. Again, the example of controlling an instinctual drive would be the desire to pull the bed covers over one's head at the sound of the morning alarm and to sleep in and not deal with the environment in an assertive manner. After a certain point, the individual has slept in beyond the point of making it to class or work on time and therefore either misses hie or her appointed schedule or arrives late. After a number of occasions of this behavior, serious consequences will probably result. The individual having this habit or condition cannot function properly. Capacity for delay in order to control instinctual drives occurs throughout the day as an individual window shops at the mall, buys groceries, or even socializes at a gathering place. Consequences for the inability to control yourself in these situations can range from running up the credit card for impulsive purchases to inappropriate social behaviors that can lead to embarrassment or more serious repercussions.

The ability to delay can also be affected by medications, illicit drugs, alcohol, or diseases of the brain. A manic-depressive illness, for example, is a condition that affects impulse control and the ability to delay instinctual drives. Certain medications such as Valium or Librium and illicit drugs can lower the ability to control behaviors by removal of the anxiety or guilt that is often associated with the delay of an action.

The ability to effectively develop a capacity for delay is also associated with the individual's ability to tolerate various frustrations and to delay pressing feelings or wishes. The inability to postpone wishes that are a hindrance to organizing and prioritizing the project at hand could be viewed as an explanation for the daydreaming or procrastination behaviors as previously discussed.

The individual who cannot delay immediate feelings and impulses about the situation he or she is in might find themselves in a comedy of errors or a tragedy. Television sitcoms make extreme humor of the individual who suddenly blurts out how he or she feels about the job to the boss. Soap operas are created from dysfunctional situations of individuals who cannot control his or her wishes or passions. A real life example of this type of situation is the Clinton-Lewinsky affair, which brought embarrassment to the office of the presidency and delayed Congress from functionally performing the work of the people.

tive individual has acquired habits that will enable him or her to ward off fatigue and distractions that interrupt organizing behaviors. For example, some individuals take rest breaks, meditate, perform stress releasing exercises, take naps, control their diet, or rely on structured systems that keep them on a path of organization (Edington & Blanchard, 1986).

The Commercialism of Organization

The great number of individuals attempting to achieve an organized lifestyle has created an enormous industry of workshops, personal planners, desk organizers, and literature all aimed at getting and keeping an individual organized. Workshops presented by "experts" give minute by minute strategies on how to organize your day and increase your productivity.

Personal planners are found in office supply stores and advertisements in the mail. Personal daily planners range from minute by minute scheduling to setting one's goals for the next 5 years. Most popular planners offer a wide variety of carrying cases and binders that house not only the day by day appointments, but offer a variety of inserts that contain a small telephone directory, finance and mileage records, phone message logs, small calculators, meeting plan worksheets, and a host of other inserts that help structure and customize one's work life.

Books with promises and methods to make an individual a more organized person fill library shelves and commercial bookstores. They range from how to manage a minute (Edington & Blanchard, 1986), up to managing your effectiveness for a lifetime (Yeager, 1991). And let's not forget such famous quotes as a "stitch in time saves nine" that remind us to take care of immediate business so that we will not waste more valuable time in the future.

The Organized Individual

From the previous definitions and exploration of organization, we might safely assume that an individual who is effective at getting started in the morning and can approach the day's tasks productively, is an individual who has learned or has acquired habits that enable him or her to quickly set aside or resolve obstructive desires or thoughts (Givens, 1993). As the day progresses, the effec-

Events Requiring Organization

Can you recall the last time you went to an orientation event, such as familiarizing yourself with a new school or college, into an internship, or a new place of employment? Can you recall the mountain of new information that was given in a seemingly short period of time, such as the location of safety equipment, bathrooms, coworkers' names, policies and procedures, the forms used by the facility, and the minute ins and outs of the facility? Can you remember feeling just a little overwhelmed at times and just a bit disorganized? For a moment try and imagine those sets of circumstances without the help of some internal or external organizing devices. Just suppose you were very ill on the day of orientation and could not comprehend the information. Or suppose someone just dumped the information in your lap and said "Look this over and if you have any questions give me a call."

The ability to orient yourself to an immediate situation gives one the ability to process information in the early stages of organization. The neurological inability to orient or the resistance of an individual to orient due to the lack of will or subconscious resistance, as previously discussed, will affect an individual's ability to organize the task at hand.

The orientation of an individual or client to a new situation should be structured to provide clear and concise information to overcome the confusion of initial information. The structuring of a situation has been demonstrated to reduce anxiety (Clark & Cross, 1986). That anxiety is an obstruction to creative thought (Kubie, 1958).

The ability to structure a situation for yourself, or the ability to provide structure for an individual needing this process, can be viewed as a necessary process to reduce anxiety. Thus, the anxiety that one may suffer over the inability to organize a particular situation may be a source of conflict that actually inhibits the organization process. The individual who suffers from this anxiety may be the individual who succumbs to chemical abuse to aid them during this period. The drug either makes them think that he or she is more competent or removes the anxiety entirely, leaving the person withdrawn from society and helpless.

In summary, one can readily identify the importance of organizational skills, and also be able to identify the causes that inhibit the ability to organize. As with any task, sometimes organizational skills need to be practiced in order to be integrated into one's repertoire of behavior. Buying the day planners is a popular and practical method to assist with organizing the daily schedule and managing time. However, the daily task and habit of actually using the planner and becoming organized may not be as easy as it initially appears. The following section is offered as a compilation of many references on time management and organizational skills.

An Organizational Task

In addition to recognizing organizational deficits, the health care professional should be able to offer exercises (tasks) that will assist the individual in creating organizational habits. The following exercise provides a general overview of the organizational process.

To initiate the organization of a situation, one must first place or sort similar articles together. Suppose you wanted to make more room in your clothes closet or clothes drawers. This task would be initiated by piling all of the clothes on the floor and sorting and placing similar clothing articles together. This is similar to conducting a brainstorming session for solutions to a health care practice related problem. Pile (write) all of the participants' ideas on a paper, and then categorize them into similar thoughts or ideas.

Second, eliminate duplicates, things that don't fit or are worn-out, or ideas that have been tried before that definitely do not work. Maybe it's time to get rid of that tie-dyed t-shirt that's two sizes too small and has been hanging around for many years. Eliminate the ideas that have been tried before that didn't work. Eliminate destructive behaviors that don't work in society.

Third, assemble what is left and take stock. Are the reasons for keeping them sound? Assess the ideas. What are the negative reasons or forces against the idea or plan? What are the positive forces for the plan? For every negative force, come up with an idea or way of overcoming the obstacle.

Fourth, construct or reconstruct storage for the articles so that space has been used efficiently. The same can be said for ideas. For ideas that have been accepted and possess a number of positive ways of overcoming obstacles, place them in a timetable or plan of action. Give them a time schedule. Place them in a structured setting so that they are easily viewed. Many day planners have a structured format for daily objectives or longer term goals. Create a place to try new behaviors. In the example of working with individuals who have addictive behaviors, the health care professional needs to help these individuals find new places where new behaviors can be used to eliminate old behaviors that contributed toward their addictions.

Finally, evaluate the results. By being organized, we should see less clutter in our closets and less complication in our lives. If one is careful and wise, the space will not be filled with more or new clutter. This space is created to enjoy life by doing the fun things that being organized has allowed.

References

Burka, J. B., & Yuen, L. M. (1983). *Procrastination: Why you do it, what to do about it.* Reading, MA: Addison Wesley.

Clark, E. N., & Cross, M. (1986). The creative clay test and an exploration of task structure. In B. J. Hemphill (Ed.), *The evaluative process in psychiatric occupational therapy.* Thorofare, NJ: SLACK Incorporated.

Edington, D. W,. & Blanchard, M. (1986). *The one minute manager gets fit: How to be fit and in shape for the rest of your life.* New York, NY: William and Morrow.

Gilbert, R. J. (1986). *Caffeine, the most popular stimulant.* New York, NY: Chelsea House.

Givens, C. J. (1993). *Superself: Doubling your personal effectiveness.* New York, NY: Simon & Shuster.

Horner, A. J. (1991). *Psychoanalytic object relations therapy.* Northvale, NJ: Jason Aronson Inc.

Kubie, L. S. (1958). *Neurotic distortion of the creative process.* Lawrence, KS: University of Kansas Press.

Maurer, J. H. (1984). *The Three Stooges book of scripts.* Secaucus, NJ: Citadel Press.

Porat, F. (1980). *Creative procrastination: Organizing your own life.* San Francisco, CA: Harper & Row.

Sapadin, L. M. & Maguire, J. (1996). *It's about time: The six styles of procrastination and how to overcome them.* New York, NY: Viking.

Simon, N. (1966). *The odd couple.* New York, NY: Random House.

Smoller, E. S. (1997). *I can't remember: Family stories of Alzheimer's disease.* Philadelphia, PA: Temple University Press.

Webster's Third New International Dictionary (1981). Springfield, MA: Merriam-Webster Inc.

Yeager, N. M. (1991). *The career doctor: Preventing, diagnosing, and curing 50 ailments that can threaten your career.* New York, NY: Wiley & Sons.

Chapter Ten

Clinical Reasoning

Threese A. Clark, MS, OTR/L

Clinical reasoning, as demonstrated by using a questioning or inquiring approach; by analyzing, synthesizing, and interpreting information; and by suggesting alternative solutions to complex issues or situations, has been identified as one of the desired components of professional behaviors, and therefore, a trait or ability which deserves attention and development. This chapter will attempt to discuss the components of reasoning and methods to promote its development. Let us begin by taking a look at the general definitions and components of reasoning.

Definition

Definitions (as found in *Webster's New World Dictionary*, 1995 edition):

Reason (noun): 1. a statement offered in explanation or justification; 2. motive for action or belief; 3. the power or process of thinking: intellect; 4. ground, cause; 5. a sane or sound mind; 6. due exercise of the faculty of logical thinking.

Reason (verb): 1. to talk with another to persuade or cause a change of mind; 2. to use the faculty of reason: think; 3. to discover or formulate by the use of reason.

The above definitions of reason as included in modern dictionaries encompass both the general meaning of reason and the act of reasoning. Reason and reasoning have long been admired and desired traits, the proclaimed center of many educational teaching experiences, and their expressed terminal learning objective. The ability to rea-

son has been acknowledged as important, if not essential, to success in most professions and occupations. Routine, non-technical jobs describe reason as "common sense," the ability to assess a repetitive, routine task and recognize variation from the norm. At this level, the ability to reason is most important to safety and successful task completion as determined by a preset standard or criteria. As tasks become more technical and job responsibilities move from the completion of established, controlled procedures to the domain of determining effectiveness, resolving problems, or creating and instituting procedures or actions, reason becomes viewed as the ability to think logically with the intent of formulating a plan based on the interpretation of available data. As such, reason and reasoning are elevated to the realm of professional behavior.

Significance

Reasoning as a professional behavior exists on multiple levels. Therefore reasoning, as a desired and necessary professional behavior, has been afforded a substantial amount of attention in recent literature and research. Since the early 1980s, a resurgence of interest in and study of reasoning has occurred. The literature resulting from this interest has generated concern and, at times, confusion. Descriptions and labels given to the process often reflect the field of origin of the study rather than identifying an approach that substantially varies from a holistic reasoning procedure. At the roots of moral reasoning, mathematical reasoning, scientific reasoning, clinical reasoning, etc., lies a basic generic process essential to all reasoning. It is vital that students, practitioners, and educators recognize and understand this fact.

Information, either formal or informal, perceived as unknown or new, is often met with some combination of anxiety, concern, fear, and/or resistance. We are most comfortable with the tried and true, the familiar and known. Even when we seek to expand our knowledge and thus our expertise, we may question our ability to function within a new or extended context. We may even be fearful of failure. Learning is most successful when the learner views him- or herself as already possessing some skills and abilities that can be used as a foundation for new experiences and learning, a building block or stepping stone. When the learner is able to identify a basic process generic to all reasoning and can identify areas in past learning or experience where he or she used the process, then he or she can envision the adaptation of those basic principles to other situations. Reasoning, in all its many disguises, is but a variation or adaptation of the basic process that is fundamental to all of its uses. Some are narrow or strictly structured, as in scientific or procedural reasoning ("the facts ma'am, just the facts"). In other applications, a broader more holistic approach is necessary as is demonstrated in clinical reasoning. Reasoning, when it has become habitual or second nature, is the cornerstone around which successful personal and professional growth occurs. A profession is only as successful and strong as its practitioners. Research has identified reasoning as one of the behaviors observed in successful practice and practitioners.

The success and future of a profession, as well as its individual practitioners, is determined by the extent to which a respect for and ability in such behaviors as reasoning and communication can be instilled in its members. Reasoning skills will define practice, determine procedures, identify competence, measure outcomes, and ensure growth. Coupled with communication skills, a necessary ability for the dissemination of the information generated, reasoning can secure the future of a profession.

Background

The ability to reason is the ability to think. Thinking consists of the ability to discover the properties and/or events affecting a situation and to identify their interplay.

It is the skill to forecast probable future occurrences and predict their effects. It is the art of interpretation and application of the data gathered (facts) for the purpose of establishing or formulating an idea or plan.

Reasoning is a combination of intelligence, understanding, and caring (Schwartz, 1991). While it was suggested earlier in this chapter that there is a basic generic process for all types of reasoning, it was also indicated that there are multiple uses for reasoning and multiple combinations of the basic components of reasoning. The appropriate combination is determined by the type of situation and the end result desired. It is these combinations which have generated the various names assigned to reasoning. Theoretical reasoning (reasoning grounded in the theory employed by a specific field or profession) differs from practical reasoning, or the reasoning exercised to solve everyday problems. A grounding in theory alone does not guarantee expert or competent practice in a profession (Mattingly, 1991). To be successful, theory must be translated into practical use. Therefore, it is essential that we follow theoretical training with practical experience. Clinical reasoning skills are required to generate from practical experience the desired outcome(s) — competent practice.

In health care professions such as occupational therapy, where it has been suggested that successful treatment must be grounded in the individual patient's experience of his illness, reasoning has been described as a process consisting of the interplay of a knowledge of disease with a frame of reference or theory as effected by experience (Mattingly, 1991). This reasoning is commonly referred to as clinical reasoning and is a desired standard for almost all health care practitioners. Clinical reasoning is the process by which clinical judgment generates clinical decisions that define and determine the procedures chosen and therefore, the service provided (Hall, 1992). The process has been described as largely tacit, highly imagistic, and deeply phenomenological (Mattingly, 1991). It is a procedure in which an intellectual process is combined with intuition, judgment, empathy, common sense, theory, experience, and foresight to produce an action plan that surpasses any strategy derived solely from logical thought, and therefore has an increased potential for success. To benefit from clinical reasoning, the practitioner must be able to visualize possibilities. The successful professional acts upon one or more of the visualized possibilities and is able to adapt or change the chosen action in answer to a response. Further modification may be required by new information or developing circumstances, and must build upon past and present experience. Clinical reasoning is a continual process that produces a "best", rather than a "right", answer for any given point in time. All decisions are and should be viewed as temporary in nature and extremely flexible.

As an example, clinical reasoning based on information gathered from the sharing of a life story could allow the individual, as well as the practitioner, to visualize outcomes and might encourage cooperation as it provided motivation. It could ensure accountability, focus the scope of services provided, and promote unique approaches to assessment. The information gathered could be used to establish unique solutions to individual problems and provide a best approach for the current situation and circumstances.

Clinical reasoning consists of several separate types of reasoning or procedures. Logical, procedural thought produces decisions, problem identification, and diagnosis. Assessing the effects of experience on an individual's roles and activities requires an interactive approach. Ongoing revision of the service or intervention as well as prediction of the future or outcome demands conditional and pragmatic reasoning that factors in contextual realities and personal characteristics. Finally, narrative reasoning produces a life story which creates an image of the future and allows all involved in the service process to focus on the steps necessary to reach that future. This holistic approach of using procedural, interactive, conditional, pragmatic, and narrative reasoning has been identified as the unique element of clinical reasoning practiced by successful health care practitioners (Neistadt, 1992; 1995). Fleming (1991) further suggested that procedural reasoning guides treatment while interactive reasoning guides therapy. Therapy (service) was felt to be imagination tempered by clinical experience and expertise.

Clinical reasoning may both limit and be limited by the setting in which the health care practitioner is found. The clinical setting may have established policies and procedures that regulate those served. It may establish the focus of service or determine the frame of reference used, and may control the resources available to the professional/practitioner. Clinical reasoning may further define these limits or it may be used to challenge them. In addition to the setting, the experience of the practitioner will affect the expression of clinical practice. The recency of use of a specific approach, the intensity with which the professional/practitioner has used a procedure, the frequency of that use, the frame of reference employed, and personal preference all influence practice (Rogers, 1991). Clinical reasoning is the instrument which can keep the professional/practitioner fresh, innovative, and invested.

General knowledge of functional deficits and treatment possibilities are insufficient to guide practice (Mattingly, 1991), and do not alone promote the evolution of the practitioner into a master clinician. Only through the practice of employing clinical reasoning does the novice become the master. Only through conversion of the beginner to the expert or master do we prepare the individual to assume key positions in the clinic, education, research, and/or professional and political community (Burke and DeBoy, 1991). Clinical reasoning is the vehicle by which this transition can be accomplished.

Nature of Clinical Reasoning

In the field of health service, the holistic model upon which clinical reasoning has been based is a more effective model than the biomedical model within which to foster the growth and effectiveness of both practice and the individual professional/practitioner. The biomedical frame of reference ignores the social and humanistic perspectives of illness (Crepeau, 1991; Fleming, 1991), often separating illness from individual experience and placing emphasis and focus on the technical. Such a focus can be both unrewarding and unsuccessful for the health care professional as well as for the patient. It has long been acknowledged that all interactions are filtered through the experiences and perceptions of the participants. While complete contextual understanding, due to its dynamic and responsive nature, is never fully realized, the attempt to understand to the best of our ability and within the timeframe of our encounter is essential to competent service delivery. This contextual understanding is, while difficult, the very essence of our clinical reasoning.

Figure 10-1 is a pictorial representation of the many aspects of the realities that must be reconciled to achieve successful intervention. This reconciliation is accomplished through clinical reasoning. The health care practitioner, the client/patient, and the contextual environment all possess strengths and weaknesses. The unique combination of these strengths and weaknesses defines the competencies of the professional/practitioner, the function or dysfunction of the client, and the individual realities of the expected living environment. The interplay of these factors defines intervention goals which, in turn, determine intervention/procedures. The evaluation and re-evaluation of the outcomes of the intervention must include the continued monitoring of the interaction of the three major players in this drama, the profes-

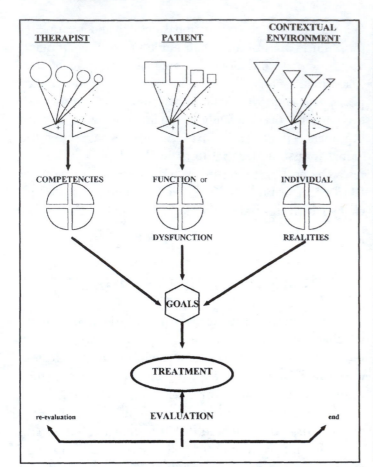

Figure 10-1. Aspects in successful intervention.

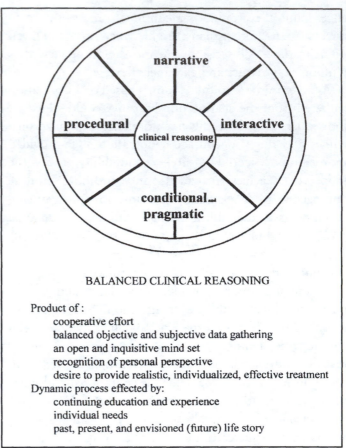

Figure 10-2. Balanced clinical reasoning.

sional/practitioner, the client, and the greater environment. This monitoring is accomplished through clinical reasoning.

Figure 10-2 depicts the balanced wheel that is essential to successful clinical reasoning. While this representation shows all spokes of the wheel to be equal, it must be understood that this does not suggest that the same attention is given to each style of reasoning at all times. The attention necessary for the balancing of the wheel may vary with the client, the stage of wellness, and the goals or priorities at any given time, as well as with the environment and the other elements involved.

The balanced wheel is always a product of a cooperative effort and is the balance of objective and subjective data. It demands an open and inquisitive approach and the recognition of the personal perspective of all players. To be effective there must be a genuine desire to provide realistic, individualized, and effective intervention. The clinical reasoning that is required to achieve this balance

is a dynamic process affected by the education, experience, needs, and goals of the individuals involved and of their past, present and envisioned future life stories. Common distortions to the wheel may be the disappearing hub (Figure 10-3a) in which the client or practitioner allows "band wagon" behavior or outside forces to take control; the enlarged hub (Figure 10-3b) where the professional/practitioner or patient has a "father (or patient) knows best" attitude resulting in over-involvement and failure to cooperate; or the misshapen wheel (Figure 10-3c) where a lack of information or an imbalance in attention to information causes inadequate intervention, unrealistic goals, and/or poor outcome.

Reasoning is not a unique behavior restricted to the professional or health care practitioner. On the contrary, it has been suggested that reasoning or thinking is what makes us human. It is the behavior that distinguishes us from other animals (even though those of us who own—oops, are owned by—our cats and dogs are not convinced

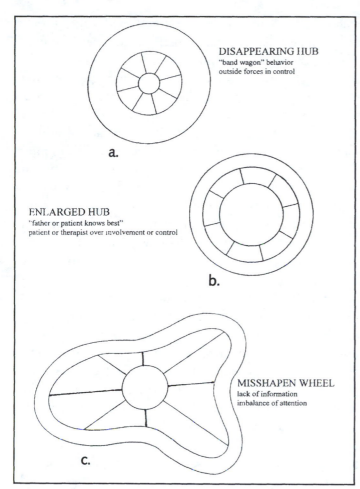

Figure 10-3. Distortions in balance.

ing to suitable decision-making and judgment is the purpose of all reasoning. Problem-solving, decision-making, and judgment are therefore the *stuff* of reasoning. Because reasoning has been defined as the power and process of thinking, we might conclude that problem-solving, decision-making, and judgment are also the end products of thinking. The goal of human thinking is to determine the best course of action in a given situation. So—how do we get there?

Development of Clinical Reasoning

Jerome Bruner suggested that humans think in two fundamentally different ways (Mattingly, 1991). Paradigmatic thinking, or propositional argument, is used when we are seeking to make sense of what we have seen and observed. It is an attempt to understand a particular in general terms. When sets of facts are seen as a general process or picture, paradigmatic thinking is being employed.

The second type of thinking is accomplished through storytelling and is known as narrative. We engage in narrative thinking when we are trying to understand a particular event or situation. It is used in an effort to comprehend the experience of the particular situation, event, or happening.

The processes used to accomplish either of these forms of thinking have been the object of a great deal of research and speculation. It is generally accepted that the process consists of four steps (Neistadt, 1992).

• Deductive reasoning allows us to ask questions and thus formulate a hypothesis (question).

• Inductive reasoning provides for the modification of the original question(s).

• Dialectical reasoning supplies an interpretation of behavior and response.

• Ethical reasoning assists with the establishment of intervention priorities that are consistent with the values of both the patient and the professional/practitioner.

Further it should be noted that these processes are approached through one of two common human perspectives (Schwartz, 1991). The justice perspective relies on the abstract concepts of truth, justice, and equality to frame solutions to dilemmas. The caring perspective emphasizes the strength of relationships.

they do not think and even plot on occasion). Some people appear to be naturally successful when employing reasoning strategies. Others improve with instruction and practice. A few appear to never quite get it, or develop the skill. No matter the background (lay person or professional/practitioner), or the level of expertise (student, novice, or master), everyone has used the basic principles of reasoning. From simple to complex, decisions are based on a degree of reasoning. This reasoning may be at such a basic level that it appears to be habit and may go unnoticed by both the performer and the observer, or it may be so complex that it appears to defy explanation. It seems to be easier to recognize poor reasoning or a lack of reasoning than it is to identify the components necessary for success.

Although the features of reasoning may be difficult to pinpoint, successful reasoning strategies are readily distinguished by their outcome. Problem-solving activity lead-

As if all of this is not challenging enough, let us add another ingredient to the mix. Thinking implies the use of intelligence. There are multiple kinds of intelligence already recognized, with more being suggested and researched. Linguistic, musical, logical-mathematical, spatial, kinesthetic, and personal intelligence have been referred to in the literature (Schwartz, 1991). Emotional IQ has even enjoyed the limelight. It is overwhelming to contemplate the nearly limitless combinations of components that are possible. A minor shift in the combination of or emphasis placed on any of the components could potentially change the process and outcome of reasoning.

Reasoning can never reach perfection because it is always based on incomplete information. It is based on information that is constantly and consistently evolving. Therefore, the best we can hope to accomplish is to make the most informed and appropriate decision possible at any given time. We must remain flexible and alert, thus ensuring the adjustment of judgment and decisions as we observe response to intervention and as we gather new information. This is the intent of clinical reasoning.

How then can we make clinical reasoning manageable and gain a degree of structure and control? How do we convince professionals/practitioners that this is not an impossible task—an exercise in futility?

Human activity is believed to be motivated and therefore, able to be explained by reason (Mattingly, 1991). Certain aspects can be standardized and some outcomes predicted. These factors help to limit possibilities and establish a general direction or goal. The ability of the human mind to attend to multiple bits and bytes of information simultaneously, to interpret those bits and bytes at numerous levels and in various combinations, or to choose to ignore the information makes clinical reasoning a uniquely human accomplishment. They are the abilities that make reasoning possible. They are skills that can be learned, sharpened, and refined. The combination of the ability to explain and predict human behavior and the capacity to interpret or set aside certain facts is perfected through practice. This is the essence of thinking and reasoning.

The acknowledgment that numerous bits of information are combined with certain known facts or beliefs suggests that reasoning and thinking have distinct parts—parts that can be broken down, studied, practiced, and perfected in smaller, less overwhelming, pieces and then recombined to produce a whole. The whole is usually greater than the sum of its parts. Facts (knowledge) pertaining to disease, function, culture, development, theory, etc. can be learned. Skills and intervention techniques can be practiced and perfected. Observation skills can be enhanced. Life experiences can be expanded. The list is endless. Learning and understanding is a lifelong task. Now superimpose upon this view the idea that there are various types of reasoning, some more structured than others. Learning principles suggest that a structured or more concrete concept is easier to understand than an abstract or unstructured one. This implies that teaching and learning of reasoning is best begun with the more concrete and structured types, possibly with diagnostic reasoning. An independent grasp of diagnostic reasoning, group interaction, cultural awareness, self-understanding, and factual knowledge can be used to build confidence and provide stepping-stones to a more complex combined use.

Diagnostic reasoning is one component of clinical reasoning (Rogers & Holm, 1991). To diagnose implies an investigation or analysis of the cause or nature of a condition, situation, or problem (Rogers & Holm, 1991). The diagnosis represents the summary of the facts presented by the client and any tests performed are tempered by observations made during the process. The facts generated are used to establish expectations, suggest severity of the problem, and predict a course of intervention. Successful intervention is expected to follow a track common to the diagnosed problem. Everyone has experienced the use of diagnostic reasoning—"rest and drink lots of liquids" or "take two aspirin and call me in the morning." Thus, medical instruction or information will seem more or less familiar. Diagnostic information and reasoning is perceived as a safe place to start—a safe foundation from which to venture forth. Diagnostic reasoning is composed of cue acquisition, hypothesis generation, cue interpretation, and hypothesis evaluation (Rogers & Holm, 1991). The ability to generate a hypothesis or question from the cues requires the ability to sense the problem. The problem must then be concisely described and precisely named. Problem definition aids in cue interpretation and makes possible the evaluation of the hypothesis. In providing treatment or intervention we may rename these steps: problem review and patient evaluation (cue acquisition), functional level performance and goal setting (hypothesis generation), re-evaluation (cue interpretation), and problem resolution or intervention outcome (hypothesis evaluation). It is not long into the use of diagnostic reasoning that the practitioner recognizes difficulties with this as a sole approach to intervention planning. The problems of clients/ patients often fail to comply with the clinical picture outlined in literature and research. It is evident that other factors influence the individual—factors that, while not necessarily medical, may have as much, if not more, effect on the outcome of intervention than do the specific facts of the problem or situation.

Diagnostic reasoning used alone will always have missing, incomplete, or inadequate data—data that is essential to the understanding of the human reaction and adaptation to events/situations. Health care professionals seek this data in an attempt to enhance their intervention planning and outcomes. The best source of information for the missing data appears to be the client. Diagnostic reasoning has laid the foundation for collaborative planning involving client input—the move to clinical reasoning. In the mutual problem-solving process, professionals/practitioners learn from their clients. To successfully do this, they must relinquish some of their authority and believe in the validity of their client's experience and perspective (Crepeau, 1991). The reward for risking this behavior is the gathering of a more complete image of the client and his or her environment. Information on beliefs, culture, values, behavior patterns, resources, support systems, reason for referral, age, sex, and past experiences not only enhances our understanding of the client but improves our ability to predict future function and provide a superior intervention plan—one with a higher probability of success. To provide relevant and meaningful intervention, the practitioner must attend on three levels: the condition, the client as a person, and the client as a social being (Fleming, 1991). This requires several modes of intellectual processing or thought. Performance problems derived from diagnostic facts are processed with logical and critical thinking. The client as a person is perceived through interactive reasoning, and possible future function is arrived at through projective thought (Schwartz, 1991). Analytical thought and instrumental measurement provides only the most basic understanding of an individual. Realistic individualized intervention is grounded in interpersonal understanding and intelligence. This inter-subjectivity demands attention to the life story of another (Crepeau, 1991). It requires that knowledge of the situation and the experience of an individual is sought to develop a more complete understanding of the person as a unique being. This information is most available through a storytelling process. The interpretation of this material is further influenced by the experience, frame of reference, personal priorities, habits, and routines of the health care professional (Rogers & Holm, 1991). Presumed functional problems must be validated through a thinking process that operates intuitively, analytically, and perceptually, as well as instru-

mentally (Fleming, 1991). This is the complex procedure known as clinical reasoning.

The end result of this clinical reasoning process is the formation of a more complete and accurate clinical image of the client. It allows for the person's assets and deficits to be tracked holistically, and may unveil available compensatory skills. Clinical reasoning as viewed from this context solicits information most easily acquired through a narrative or storytelling approach. Narratives give meaningful structure to life over time (Mattingly, 1991). It pictures the individual as a larger temporal whole and, as mentioned earlier in this chapter, facilitates the understanding of a particular case rather than providing a general description of a condition or event. This broader approach fosters organization of the individual's life as an entirety, assisting with the establishment of a more realistic set of priorities and decreasing the risk of noncompliance (Neistadt, 1995). Narratives decrease the danger of missing activities of primary importance. Clients may answer only direct questions during a formal evaluation for fear that their stories are of little or no interest to the professional/practitioner. Narratives encourage the sharing of this information and allow for alignment and realignment within the interaction. The narrative may even dictate the mood and agenda of the session (Crepeau, 1991). It can be used to elicit active cooperation and commitment. There is the possibility, almost the certainty, that irrelevant information may also be obtained. It is the skill of the professional/practitioner that enables him or her to sort this information and use narrative effectively. This skill can be learned and perfected, and mastery can be obtained only through experience and practice.

Levels of Development

There are multiple levels of mastery along the road to obtaining clinical reasoning skills. Masters have been described as those professionals/practitioners who have a common identifiable ideology, a highly developed knowledge base, and a set of essential, individualized behaviors that have been expanded through extensive, varied experience (Burke & DePoy, 1991). The master practitioner's skill lays in the implementation of interventions, and five levels of mastery have been identified (Slates & Cohen, 1991; Neistadt, 1995). These levels in order of development are: novice, advanced beginner, competent professional/practitioner, proficient professional/practitioner, and expert or excellent (master) practitioner.

• The *novice* is the new graduate or health care professional expanding skills into an area previously not experienced. This practitioner feels most comfortable using the "rules". He or she remains in the safe objective arena, leaving treatment and planning generally context-free.

• The *advanced beginner* starts to consider additional cues. These cues remain largely objective. While the advanced beginner is able to assess behavior, he or she is unable to attach meaning. At this level intervention and intervention planning continue to be situation- and context-free. The professional/practitioner is unable to determine priorities and fails to perceive the entire picture.

• The *competent health care professional* is able to individualize intervention. He or she can identify relevant facts and is able to prioritize. However, the competent practitioner still lacks the experience that allows for flexibility and creativity. Therefore, opportunities to revise plans and improve outcomes are often missed.

• The *proficient professional/practitioner* perceives situations as wholes. He or she demonstrate a sense of direction and vision that is derived from considering options. Modification of intervention and approach appear to be automatic.

• The *expert* is the professional/practitioner who shifts rules to the background. He or she possesses an intuitive grasp of a situation. The expert or excellent (master) practitioner employs an interaction of intellect, emotion, and personality that results in adaptability to environmental challenges. This individual is motivated to use nontraditional approaches to achieve desired outcomes. The expert uses habitual and automatic knowledge. He or she is often described as someone who can think "on their feet" —as one who thinks while doing (Mattingly, 1991).

Of the two characteristics of the highest level of mastery, excellence and expertise, expertise is the more desirable and more growth-sustaining. Excellence is a public entity. Excellent behavior is recognized by comparing action to a set of predetermined and accepted public standards. Excellence is the public recognition of mastery. The excellent professional/practitioner has vision, is innovative, and strives to become better (Burke & DePoy, 1991). Expertise (mastery), the highest level of performance, is more private. It is individual accomplishment. Mastery consists of a personal knowing—a confidence in one's action, experience, and thinking that does not rely on public recognition. The master health care professional has personal characteristics of creativity, commitment,

and intelligence. He or she employs an individual creative reasoning style that is sustained without the need for public acclaim. This is the highest level of attainment; one that may never be totally achieved as the master forever strives to climb higher and learn more. As the practitioner advances through the levels of practice, the gap between what one knows and what one can say or explain about what he knows grows. Practice/intervention becomes "thinking in action" (Mattingly, 1991). This is the very phenomenon that makes teaching clinical reasoning difficult. However, as this is a behavior that is essential to successful practice, development cannot be left to chance.

How quickly the concepts related to beginning clinical reasoning are understood and to what degree they are internalized may be influenced by a number of factors. For instance, the age and life experience of the learner may have a positive or negative effect on both the speed with which the ideas are understood and the depth of that understanding. The older individual or the one with a larger repository of life experiences is often able to link the concepts and behaviors that constitute clinical reasoning to successes or failures experienced in other situations. These experiences can act as building blocks and provide some degree of reassurance that the learner is capable of performing the desired behavior. The presence or absence of role models throughout the individual's life also has an effect. Role models do not need to be from the profession/occupation being pursued. An individual from home, school, church, community, or even history who has demonstrated success with using clinical reasoning to make decisions in his or her life can motivate and encourage others to attempt to behave in a similar manner. A mentor who assists the learner through beginning attempts to understand and use the concept is also of great importance. The mentor must be someone who is able to assess where the learner is, accept their successes and failures unconditionally, and be willing to see the mentee outgrow them. At the novice level, learners should demonstrate a questioning of facts, ideas, and situations. They should seek to expand their understanding of medical conditions and facts, environmental influences, cultures, values, and lifestyles unfamiliar to them. They should begin to form opinions and ideas on how their observations may be interpreted and risk sharing these ideas with others to further expand and refine their knowledge. Flexibility, open-mindedness, curiosity, and an ability to observe are the behaviors that will support the development of clinical reasoning skills.

Intermediate clinical reasoning behaviors should begin to emerge with laboratory classes and clinical experiences. The learner should now begin to use the factual knowledge that has been obtained to generate a hypothesis that can be used for treatment planning and intervention. A willingness to listen to and act upon constructive criticism and suggestions will serve them well. This is the stage at which theory and facts begin to be used in the real world of practice. A critical and honest assessment of his or her success is the individual's most powerful tool for fostering growth. At this level, the influence of the contextual and situational environment upon the treatment planning process and its success should begin to be integrated.

Advanced clinical reasoning skills begin to develop after the completion of all academic and clinical requirements, and the individual is now ready to enter his or her chosen field as a novice health care professional. They will begin to use their skills in clinical reasoning with the responsibility for treatment success being, for the first time, theirs. They will have to recognize the need for supervision and be willing to seek it out. The responsibility for professional growth is theirs. As they become secure in this new role and gain experience, they can begin to improve and perfect their clinical reasoning skills. The degree to which the health care professional is able to develop the ability to reason clinically and think critically is an important determinant of his or her skill as a service provider, and of the success of the treatment and intervention delivered. The effect on the quality of life enjoyed by their clients is the ultimate consideration.

Conclusion

How do we grow, develop, and acquire this important professional behavior? Guided observation and case studies can be used to enhance cue acquisition, hypothesis generation, cue interpretation, and hypothesis evaluation. One can learn to recognize relevant data and distinguish subjective from objective fact. Role play and debate can broaden response choices for intervention planning and situational conduct. Connected learning offers the opportunity to understand the application of fact and technique in various settings and situations. Multiple causes for and explanations of events can be introduced and explored. Cerebral data files can be established, expanded, amended, and rearranged, allowing for unlimited combinations of facts and ideas. Clinical observation and role models or mentors can assist with making the transition from theory to the real world of work or to expand effec-

tiveness within that world. Physical, social, cultural, and environmental realities can be introduced under controlled conditions where support decreases the risk and fear of failure. The highly individualized nature of treatment, intervention planning, and provision can be introduced in a guided manner. These approaches can be used for formal or informal life-long learning.

Methods and Ideas

The following exercise is used in our curriculum at Mount Aloysius College, and is designed to attempt to establish a connection between all theory and practice courses. The activity is designed to establish an appreciation of the interconnectedness of fact, practice, and personal experiences and to explore how these factors effect and are affected by various situations, events and conditions. This assignment has been dubbed "The Phantom Citizen". In the Lifespan Development courses, learners work in small groups to create a citizen, from birth to death. The only restrictions on their creation is that the person may not have a major disease or disability and that he or she must live to a normal life expectancy of 75 to 80 years. The person created must experience all of the normal developmental milestones and must have a social, educational, cultural, economic, vocational, and religious background. Family and community factors and living conditions must be included. In subsequent practice classes, the citizen is given a major disease or disability that corresponds to the area of practice being covered: pediatrics, psychosocial, adult rehabilitation, or geriatric practice. The citizen's life is altered to reflect the effects of the disease or condition, given his or her original characteristics and circumstances, and outlines his or her reaction and response to the situation. Each citizen and alteration is presented to the class in both oral and written format. The learners are encouraged to make their presentations interesting and complete. They may videotape actual places, role play the citizen, or present their case in any manner that will accomplish their goal. By completion of the program and graduation, each citizen will have been constructed and reconstructed in five various situations. Learners will have a catalogue with a minimum of 30 representative citizens (six citizens per class times five alterations) who were created and then through clinical reasoning were altered, upon which to draw from to understand the holistic nature of clients and intervention provision and the effects of contextual occurrences upon the process.

Another learning activity used to foster the development and understanding of clinical reasoning and to provide beginning experience in its use is the "How to Host a Clinical Reasoning Experience" game. Learners are furnished with a very brief clinical picture of an imaginary or real client. They are given several weeks to develop long-term goals based only on the information provided. No assumptions are made, only the facts provided are to be used to determine goals. A list of missing information or "would like to know statements" may be made but not used. The set of goals is submitted to the facilitator. Accuracy of the goals is not the concern, therefore, there is no right or wrong answer to this part of the exercise. One week in advance of the second step, a role play situation, learners are chosen to be the players. Each person is provided with a basic personality sketch of his or her character. Some information is designated as "must share" during the experience, while other information may or may not be made known at the discretion of the participant, or can be determined by the direction that the role play may take. At intervals during the experience the facilitator will give additional information to the players. This information may tell the person more about his or her character, may give information on another character, or may outline a contextual situation to be included. The only rule for the experience is that if asked a direct question, the player must answer honestly based on the information he or she has been given concerning the character. If no information is available to answer the question, fabrication is fair. Characters may include but are not limited to: client, parent/spouse or significant other, sibling or child, nurse, doctor, PT, OT, social worker, case manager, dietitian, insurance representative, referral source personnel, etc. At the end of the role play experience small groups are established. These groups formulate a treatment and intervention plan based on all the information now available. They compare this plan to the original list of goals as presented by team members during the first stage of the assignment and prioritize them. Groups are given 2 weeks to complete their plan. At the end of the 2-week preparation time, groups are required to present and defend their choice of goals and the priority with which they will be addressed. The format for the presentation is that common to debate team meets. Clinical reasoning based on contextual and factual information is the emphasis of this exercise.

Additional Assignments

A cultural tree assignment requires the learner to find and explain a symbol from a culture or group other than their own and to present the meaning of that practice, symbol, or belief to his or her associates. An object representative of the practice or belief is made to decorate the cultural (not Christmas) tree that is displayed in the department's lobby during the holiday season.

The learner will be exposed to actual practice situations during clinical course experiences. A seminar to reflect upon and share these experiences is a requirement related to all of these courses.

The College requires that all senior students participate in the Capstone Seminar and write an integrated paper designed to provide a final synthesis of learning, values, experiences, and beliefs. The current topical question for this seminar is "What does it mean to be a citizen of the world?"

All of these experiences can be adapted for environments outside of a formal classroom setting (e.g., journal/cultural experience club(s), case study discussions, grand rounds, etc.).

Other Ideas and Sources

Other methods of fostering the development of clinical reasoning are narrative reporting, interviewing, and backward processing where the outcomes of treatment are presented (two similar cases with decidedly different results) and the learner tries to determine the reasons for difference in outcome.

Additional resource information may be found in Susan Fowler Woodring's audio tape series titled *Mentoring: How to Foster Your Career's Most Crucial Relationships* published in 1992 by CareerTrack Publications; in Robert J. Sternberg's book *Successful Intelligence: How Practical and Creative Intelligence Determine Success in Life*; and in *Emotional Intelligence: Why It Can Matter More Than IQ* written by Daniel Goleman and published by Bantam Books in 1995.

Clinical reasoning practice in game format can be found in the computer programs produced by Seria titled: *Incredible Machines, More Incredible Machines,* and *Incredible Machines III.*

References

Burke, J. P., & DePoy, E. (1991). An emerging view of mastery, excellence, and leadership in occupational therapy practice. *American Journal of Occupational Therapy, 45,* 1027-1032.

Crepeau, E. B. (1991). Achieving intersubjective understanding: Examples from an occupational therapy treatment session. *American Journal of Occupational Therapy , 45,* 1016-1025.

Fleming, M. H. (1991). Clinical reasoning in medicine compared with clinical reasoning in occupational therapy. *American Journal of Occupational Therapy, 45,* 988-996.

Fleming, M. H. (1991). The therapist with the three-track mind. *American Journal of Occupational Therapy, 45,* 1007-1014.

Hall, L., Robertson, W., & Turner, M. A. (1992). Clinical reasoning process for service provision in the public school. *American Journal of Occupational Therapy, 46,* 927-936.

Mattingly, C. (1991). The narrative nature of clinical reasoning. *American Journal of Occupational Therapy, 45,* 998-1005.

Mattingly, C. (1991). What is clinical reasoning. *American Journal of Occupational Therapy, 45,* 979-986.

Mattingly, C., & Fleming, M. F. (1994). *Clinical reasoning: Forms of inquiry in a therapeutic practice.* Philadelphia, PA: F. A. Davis.

Mattingly, C., & Gillette, N. (1991). Anthropology, occupational therapy, and action research. *American Journal of Occupational Therapy, 45,* 972-978.

Neistadt, M. E. (1992). The classroom as clinic: Applications for a method of teaching clinical reasoning. *American Journal of Occupational Therapy, 46,* 814-819.

Neistadt, M. E. (1996). Teaching strategies for the development of clinical reasoning. *American Journal of Occupational Therapy, 50,* 676-684.

Neistadt, M. E., & Athens, A. (1996). Analysis of the orthopedic content in occupational therapy curriculum from a clinical reasoning perspective. *American Journal of Occupational Therapy, 50,* 669-675.

Rogers, J. C., & Holm, M. B. (1991). Occupational therapy diagnostic reasoning: A component of clinical reasoning. *American Journal of Occupational Therapy, 45,* 1045-1053.

Schwartz, K. B. (1991). Clinical reasoning and new ideas on intelligence: Implications for teaching and learning. *American Journal of Occupational Therapy, 45,* 1033-1037.

Slates, D. Y., & Cohen, E. S. (1991). Staff development through analysis of practice. *American Journal of Occupational Therapy, 45,* 1038-1044.

Webster's Third New International Dictionary (1981). Springfield, MA: Merriam-Webster Inc.

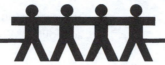

Chapter Eleven

Supervisory Process

Sherry L. Pfister,
AAS, COTA/L

Barbara Tennent-Ponterio,
MS, OTR/L

Think back to your memories as a child or picture your own children. The parent says to the child, "How big are you?" The child stretches out tiny arms a short amount and proudly exclaims, "Sooo big!" The parent moves the child's arms further apart and says, "You are *this big*."

Imagine this same child as an 8-year-old little leaguer. The parent teaches and then practices with the child how to throw a fast ball. Repeating directions and making small corrections in throwing technique are made throughout the process. All the while, the child soaks up the information and support, believing that the parent is the smartest mom or dad on Earth! After the championship game, the parent hoists the child up on a broad shoulder and cries out, "Yeah, that's my kid!" Finally, visualize the child turned into a young adult. After years of helping with homework, revoking of driving privileges, and listening to the heartbreak of puppy loves, the parent rejoices that graduation day has arrived. The parent, realizing that it is time to let go, embraces the child and says, "I'm so proud of you. You're all grown up!"

This is what the truly effective supervisory process is about, the ability to assist another person to become competent and confident. Although parent and child are not equal in knowledge, control, or power, there is the hope and expectation that the child will learn the skills needed to grow into a responsible adult. Hopefully, the parent also learns to adapt his or her behaviors and approaches as the child matures. By doing so, the parent gains insight into his or her own skills. The roles are interdependent— one is not fully functional without the other. The parent is not a parent without the child, a child is not parented without a parent.

Supervisory Process Defined

According to the *American Heritage Dictionary* (1976), to supervise is "to direct and inspect the performance of work or workers." Depending on the context, supervise can also mean to manage, control, or oversee. Although these definitions are accurate and acceptable, they are seemingly one-sided and do not portray the two-sided exchange involved in an effective supervisory relationship.

The Goal of This Chapter

It is the goal of this chapter to help further define what an effective supervisory process includes and to enhance supervision in everyday practice.

Supervision in professional practice should include shared, reciprocal exchanges in which the *supervisory participants,* those involved in the working relationship, become interdependent. The key terms are *shared* and *reciprocal.* Consider the following two scenarios that could have come from the popular television show, *Melrose Place.*

SCENARIO 1

Amanda Woodward, the Supervisor: Let's get those ad files done now!

Allison Parker, the Supervisee: But I still have to see Mr. Jones about...

Amanda: I said now, not tomorrow! Get to it.

SCENARIO 2

After the owner of the agency resigns suddenly because Amanda was blackmailing him, the new owner fires Amanda and replaces her with Billy, the "good guy"...

Billy, the Supervisor: We need to get those ad files updated and organized into alphabetical order by the end of today.

Allison Parker, the Supervisee: But I still need to see Mr. Jones about the ad campaign that he requested. Do you agree that Mr. Jones is a priority?

Billy: How long will it take you to do that?

Allison: Probably until the end of the day, but first, I'll ask Chris to come and help out with the files.

In order for the supervisory process to work effectively, the participants involved must share information constantly by giving and receiving feedback. The task to be completed is clearly defined in terms of deadline (end of today), specifics are clarified (updated and organized), tasks are mutually prioritized (Mr. Jones a priority), and each listens to the other openly. When the supervisory process is effective, then growth of knowledge, performance skills, and a resultant higher quality of product or service will take place as the participants confer. The remainder of the chapter will focus on guiding the learner from acquiring basic supervisory concepts to a mastery of professional supervisory skills.

The Changing Supervision Focus

The number of duties performed by health care professionals has dramatically increased under corporate downsizing and "do more with less" philosophies. Supervision in today's health care market has become increasingly important. The number of assistants or paraprofessionals in many fields has increased in an attempt to provide services while at the same time keeping costs under control. Any health care professional may find him- or herself quickly thrust into the supervisory role. In this instance, professionals may throw up their hands in frustration and mutter, but they didn't teach us that in school!

Learning Supervision

Where does one *first* learn how to supervise and be supervised? Most of us learn from watching our caretakers at home, our neighbors, and community leaders (for example teachers, Brownie leaders, band directors, coaches, etc.). Who supervised the morning routine at home, the yard work, the camping trip, or the kickball game? The answers could vary from mom to dad, to the Brownie or Cub leader, to yourself. How did the leaders know how to supervise the game? They watched the role models around them and learned to determine what needed to be done, which person was best for the job, what type of behaviors were expected, and how their responses affected the relationships and/or outcome.

It is much the same with the supervisory working relationship. Each supervisory participant must first identify his or her personal needs, the needs of the other supervisory participant, and the needs of the clients or customers being served. Each participant can then begin to prioritize and develop a strategy to meet each need effectively.

Identification of Needs

How are needs identified? The first step is to understand the inherent uniqueness as well as the similarities of each individual. Prior to 1970, the workplace consisted mainly of white, married males who were raised and worked in their local region (Jameson & O'Mara, 1991). This group of workers were highly similar in background, values, and beliefs. Today, concepts like diversity, ethnicity, disabilities, and family values need to be considered. All of these and more are reflected in the changing workplace.

As the demographics of the workplace change, each person brings into the supervisory relationship an increasingly varied background, personal history, values, and cultural system. In effect, the first step is getting to know oneself and others.

Similar Needs

Levinson (1962) identified that all people have common needs when entering a workplace. Both supervisor and supervisee want to feel supported by others, to feel close to others, to be guided, and to feel safe and protected within this process. Each supervisory participant has the expectation, either conscious or unconscious, that these needs will be fulfilled in the workplace. When these needs are satisfied, the supervisory process becomes more effective. When these needs are not considered, decreased motivation and efficiency will be a natural result.

Expectations of Behavior

There are specific techniques and skills that need to be evident in the work performance of the supervisee. These generally encompass duties included in the job description as well as the professional standards of practice within the particular profession. Skill expectations such as performing a transfer, giving an inoculation, etc. are generally definitive and explicit.

Less clearly defined expectations of behavior can be called *individual standards*. What an individual believes to be important behaviors may or may not be equally important to the other involved in the supervisory process. For example, most people would agree that arriving at work on time is an expected behavior in most work situations. However, one can ask the question, how often is it okay to be late for work? Each supervisor and supervisee would have a differing perception of acceptable behavior. For example, Supervisor #1, Gabriel, may think that being 5 minutes late is an acceptable behavior if it occurs only once or twice a week. Supervisor #2, Damian, may expect daily promptness, no excuses. Other individual standards may include behaviors such as how much initiative is expected, how one is expected to respond to changes, what one does with "down" time, etc.

Each individual has an innate way of reacting or behaving in any given situation that can be called a *behavioral trait* or *style* (TRANSACT Inc., 1987). This is a person's *first* reaction to a situation. It has a genetic basis and remains steady throughout one's lifetime (Chess & Thomas, 1977; 1986). Studies by Rothbart and Derryberry (1981) seem to indicate that one's behavioral style is not affected by age or cultural diversity.

Specific behavioral traits may either foster or hinder the supervisory process. These include:
- How one reacts to new situations
- How intensely an individual reacts to a situation
- Adaptability to changes
- Persistence to complete tasks
- Positive or negative degree of one's reactions

Table 11-1 indicates the impact of each behavioral style and the potential implications of these traits in a clinical situation.

If you complete the Behavioral Style Questionnaire in Table 11-2, you can gain a clearer understanding of your own reactions in a work situation. Ask a friend or family member to also rate how they believe you react. This will give you a clearer perception of your behaviors.

Predicting Behavior

If supervisory participants can identify behavioral traits in themselves and others, they can then predict how the other participant may behave in any given situation. There are many ways to predict how an individual may behave (TRANSACT Inc., 1987). These include interviews, and skilled observation. Questionnaires are the easiest method of identifying an individual's behavioral traits. Once each supervisory participant identifies his or her own behavioral style and compares it with the other participants', he or she can begin to understand how these traits affect their interactions within the supervisory process.

How Behavioral Traits Affect the Supervisory Process

The supervisor and supervisee have individual standards and behavioral traits that vary. By using collaboration within the supervisory process, less bias, stereotyping, prejudice, and power struggles are noted. For example, when presented with a new policy or procedure, some supervisees may approach this new occurrence with open arms. In other words, the behavioral style of these individuals is an *approach orientation* to new things. Other supervisees may question the need for a new policy, ask many questions about how the policy was developed, etc. Because it takes these individuals a while to warm up to new things, they have a more *withdrawn orientation* to new situations. If both the supervisor and supervisee share an approach orientation when confronted with a change or new idea, it could be assumed that they would make a team effort. This is due to the "matching" of expectations (i.e., individual standards). Conversely, if one participant has an approach orientation and the other has a more withdrawn orientation to newness, subsequent problems or confrontations could occur because expectations are not matched.

Table 11-1

COMMON BEHAVIORAL TRAITS

Normal Trait Continuums*

Withdraw.........................Approach

Our individual reactions to new things can range from those who initially take a more cautious approach (withdraw) to those who initially have a more accepting orientation (approach).

Slow Adaptability.........................Easy Adaptability

Our individual reactions to changes can range from those who need time to adapt to situations (slow adaptability) to those who embrace change with ease (easy adaptability).

Low Intensity.........................High Intensity

How intense our reactions are to a stimulus can range from those who have extremely mild-mannered reactions (low intensity) to those who have very strong, intense reactions (high intensity) .

Negative.........................Positive

Our initial reaction to a stimulus can range from a negative response to a positive response.

Low Persistence.........................High Persistence

The length of time an activity is pursued can range from those who may need a "push" to complete tasks (low persistence) to those who will are capable of prolonged, sustained effort (high persistence).

Impact in Clinic

How we react to a new stimulus can include new clients, new coworkers, new treatment techniques, unfamiliar equipment, and new procedures and policies.

How we react to change can include our reactions to the frequency and intensity of changes in client conditions, changes in scheduling, changes in work hours, changes in staffing, and any changes we need to make in response to the therapeutic relationship with clients.

How intensely we react within a clinic situation can impact the communication process, our reactions to stress, death and dying, and the therapeutic relationship with clients.

Whether we initially react in a positive spirit or a negative spirit can influence our outlook.

How persistent we are can affect our ability to problem solve, manage time, and our reliability.

* Based on the work of Thomas & Chess (1977,1986), Lerner & Lerner (1987), and Buss & Plomin (1984), the behavioral traits of an individual can be identified. Each of us falls somewhere along the continuum, and anywhere along the continuum is "normal".

What Happens When Expectations Differ?

How we expect others to behave is based on our behavioral style. We may place a label on behaviors that may differ from our own, and make a *value judgment* based upon how we would *like* the other person to behave. For example:

Mary is the immediate supervisor for Anna. Mary is always the first one to arrive at work and the last one to leave. Mary says, "I can't bear to leave my desk unless all the work is cleared off."

Anna usually rushes to work each day, barely punching in on time. While Anna does her work thoroughly and completely, she sometimes waits until the last minute to finish and her desk is piled high with papers, brochures, and empty coffee cups.

While Mary has no complaints about the quality of Anna's work, she believes that "If Anna wasn't so disorganized and lazy, she could get a lot more work done. Thank God I'm the boss!"

While Anna has no particular complaints about the supervision that she receives from Mary, she feels that,

Table 11-2

BEHAVIORAL STYLE QUESTIONNAIRE

For each section, circle the number of the scenario that comes closest to describing your reaction in most situations.

Section I

1. It takes me a while to adapt to change. I prefer routine and structure. I like to sit back and think things through before I make a decision. I don't like having demands placed on me. It takes time for me to get used to things.

2. I love change... the more the better. As a matter of fact, I'd probably be bored if things always stayed the same. If changes don't come to me, I'll probably look for a way to do things differently.

Section II

1. If I see something that I am unfamiliar with, my first reaction is extreme interest. If it's new, I want to experience it. I feel comfortable meeting new people and doing new things.

2. If I am exposed to something new, I like to have the time to adjust. Just because it's new, doesn't mean that it's better. Sometimes I get nervous when I'm expected to meet new people or learn something I'm unfamiliar with.

Section III

1. I could be considered mild-mannered. Although I may have very intense feelings, it may not show outwardly. I'm not one to wear my heart on my sleeve.

2. I feel things intensely and it probably shows outwardly. When I'm happy, I laugh out loud. If I'm sad, you can probably see it on my face.

Section IV

1. If I'm really interested in something, I keep at it until it's completed. Very little distracts me when I'm on a roll.

2. It seems there's never enough time to get my work done. I get distracted by so many things, that someone else may need to remind me to do this or that.

Section V

1. I have a tendency to see the glass as half-full instead of half-empty. Inwardly, my first reaction to things is very positive.

2. Although others may not see it, my first reaction to things is generally less than hopeful. Things can and do go wrong.

Scoring: Although this questionnaire is not an exact measurement of behavioral functioning, you can get an indication as to where you may fall on the trait continuum.

Section I (Adaptability): This section describes how you initially respond to changes.

If you chose #1, you have a more cautious approach to change. In a clinic situation you may feel pressured if asked to make decisions very quickly or if the work pace is fast.

In an unstructured environment, you may need to create your own routines even though they may be unusual. You may also need to temper your cautiousness with deliberate risk-taking.

If you chose #2, you have an easy approach to change. In a clinic situation, changes in scheduling, etc. don't really bother you. You may feel frustrated or stifled if your work is very routine. You may need to ask to work on special projects and assignments to lessen the chance of boredom.

Section II (Approach/Withdraw): This section describes how you react to new situations.

If you chose #1, you have a more go-get-it approach to anything new. In clinic situations, this could be a strength if you can share your thoughts and ideas with others. You may want to volunteer to run new pilot programs or participate in research studies.

If you chose #2, you have a more cautious approach to new things. In a clinic situation, this can be a real strength when weighing out the consequences and outcomes of new techniques or programs.

Section III (Intensity): This section describes how intensely you react to things.

If you chose #1, you have a lower intensity of reaction to things. In a clinic situation, you have an approach that can be very calming. You will need to have good communication skills with supervisors and others since they may not know what you are feeling.

If you chose #2, you have a higher intensity of reaction to things. In a clinic situation, you may have an enthusiasm that is contagious. You will need to do some self-monitoring of your body language when dealing with difficult situations.

Section IV (Persistence): This section describes how persistent you are in activities.

If you chose #1, you have a higher persistence to get the job done. You stick with a task until it is completed. You may need to set time limits on certain tasks for time management reasons.

If you chose #2, you have a lower persistence for completing tasks. You may want to break tasks into smaller parts for time management in order to complete tasks.

Section V (Negative/Positive Mood): This section describes the degree to which you respond to life events in a negative or positive spirit.

If you chose #1, you have a more positive orientation to things.

If you chose #2, you have a more negative orientation to things. You may need more encouragement than someone on the other end of the continuum.

"If Mary would just chill out and stop expecting every-one to be so perfect, then everyone would feel less stress. Too bad I'm not the boss!"

If Mary and Anna had a clearer understanding of how their behavioral traits affect each other, they could avoid placing negative labels (value judgments) on the other's very normal, but very different, behavioral styles. Then Mary would realize that Anna's lower persistence level does not make her lazy. Conversely, Anna would realize that Mary's higher persistence level does not make her a perfectionist. Both Mary and Anna could then see that the relationship is not about control, but rather an appreciation that individual characteristics contribute to make the whole.

Responding to Differing Expectations

While one may not be able to control his or her *innate* behavioral style, that person can change how those traits are *expressed* (TRANSACT Inc., 1987) within the supervisory process. Suppose that you are an individual who reacts loudly and intensely in stressful situations. Your patient does something that makes you feel angry. Do you yell at the patient? Of course not, you have to learn to control the outward intensity of your feeling. You can still *feel* angry but your expression of it must be modified because of the expectations of the clinic situation.

Supervisory Qualities

What skills or qualities does the supervisory participant need in order to modify his or her expression of behavioral traits? Recognition and development of the following specific qualities will aid both participants within the supervisory relationship. This allows both supervisory participants to adapt how they express and how they accept their behavioral styles.

These qualities include flexibility, attitude, trust, respect, support, and conflict management.

Flexibility

Many believe that change is one of the most stressful and resisted processes that employees must deal with. Flexibility allows for ongoing change within the supervisory process. As one grows within a given health care field, changes can occur in role performance, distribution of duties, and acceptance of responsibility for risk taking. Power struggles result when change either does or does not occur as expected. Flexibility allows for that power struggle to be held in a collaborative versus adversarial manner. Consider the following illustration:

Chris has been employed as a health care worker for the past 5 years. She is described as a real go-getter. Chris feels that she has a clear understanding of her job responsibilities and would like to assist her supervisor in scheduling and management duties. Chris asks her supervisor for an increased level of role responsibility. The supervisor hesitates to allow Chris this responsibility because she feels that the department is running smoothly at this time.

Both Chris and her supervisor need to adapt their behaviors to a more flexible approach. Chris may need to step back and decide on only *one* additional duty to assume. The supervisor may need to take a risk to allow Chris the room to grow professionally. Although this may not be comfortable for them, they accept individual differences, allow new skill areas to be developed, and turn areas of weakness into strengths.

Review your completed Behavioral Style Questionnaire in the areas of Adaptability (Section I), Approach/ Withdraw (Section II), and Persistence (Section IV). Do you think that flexibility is a quality that you will need to more fully develop?

Attitude

One of the most global aspects of the supervisory process is each participant's attitude. For example, consider the following statement made by a supervisor, "The value of unions in health care facilities is questionable." Would you say that this supervisor has a positive or negative attitude toward unions? Depending on *your* attitude toward unions, you may perceive the supervisor as having *either* a negative or a positive attitude.

Read the following list of topics. Would you say you have a positive or a negative attitude toward these?

- Your job
- Your family
- Government
- Pets
- A person with AIDS

An individual's attitude can be either positive or negative in any given situation. The perception of whether another person's attitude is positive or negative is based on personal beliefs and values. *How we express* our attitude can also be perceived by others as being either positive or negative.

List five ways that characterize how someone may express a negative attitude (e.g., complain loudly).
1.
2.
3.
4.
5.

List five ways that characterize how someone may express a positive attitude (e.g., smile quietly).
1.
2.
3.
4.
5.

If you compare your list with others you may find a vast range of ways different people express attitudes. Positive attitude expression may run the gamut from smiling quietly to talking exuberantly. Negative attitude expression can range from no outward expression to yelling.

In today's health care market, supervisory participants have little time to devote to trying to change another's attitudes. Each participant in the supervisory process needs to recognize that the other may express his or her attitudes differently. Communication is essential in order to validate one's perception of another's attitude expression.

Based on your behavioral style in Section V (Negative/Positive Mood), do you think that learning to express yourself in a more positive way is something that you need to develop?

Trust

Trust takes time to develop. It occurs when each supervisory participant relies upon the other to perform obligations as agreed upon. Each participant in the supervisory process must be aware of what standards of practice guide their profession. Both participants must be aware of the need to maintain competence within their profession. One of the best ways to do this is to keep an ongoing supervisory log that includes what skills have been developed and how competence was measured. For example, a supervisee may observe the supervisor complete an interview of a patient to gather baseline information. The supervisee concurrently documents pertinent information gathered during the interview. The supervisor and supervisee compare their results to determine how similar or different their individual results were. Together, the participants have predetermined that if 95% of the infor-

mation gathered is similar, then the supervisee is competent and can be expected to perform the task independently. The supervisee then records, in the log, the date, skill achieved, and level of competence attained. An increased level of trust develops as both participants share expectations of performance.

Compare your completed Behavioral Style Questionnaire with the completed questionnaire of someone you trust. What areas, if any, are similar? Has this contributed to shared expectations of behavior?

Respect

Respect is considering another person's point of view. In the supervisory relationship, each participant must be able to adapt his or her feelings to a variety of situations. This allows for negotiation with other clinicians, departments, and officials within the facility for an overall positive representation of the team or department. One does not get respect by shouting, "Do it my way!" but rather, one earns it by proving that he or she is competent and can effectively meet the needs of all team members. Discussion and communication with each other is necessary to accurately assess the other's individual behaviors and feelings.

Look at Section II (Approach/Withdraw) on the behavioral questionnaire and compare your response with someone who reacts differently from yourself. Do you respect their difference of behavior? Do you believe that they should react more like you? How do you express your reaction?

Support

Support within the supervisory process continues to build on the trust and respect aspects by reinforcing the performance of the other participant. Support from the supervisor may include complimenting the supervisee on a job well done, reinforcing a difficult decision, or being human when family emergencies strike. It is through these seemingly small gestures that the supervisory relationship is strengthened. In the same way in which the supervisor supports the supervisee, the supervisee should also support the supervisor.

Look at Section III (Intensity) on your Behavioral Style Questionnaire. Would your behavioral style affect the way you express support to another person? Is there anything that you may need to change about the way you express your emotions?

Conflict Management

Conflict management is often seen as negative, but it is a paradoxical phenomenon. While we all hope that conflict never arises, realistically, it always does! What causes it? Time pressure, difficult people, varying behavioral traits, etc. How should the participants in the supervisory relationship cope?

First of all, communicate with each other! Dissension is caused by talking behind another's back and not directly confronting the issue. Many people tend to avoid conflict at all costs. However, avoiding conflict can result in a poor perception of management, inefficiency, low motivation, unacceptable behaviors, and loss of good employees. On the other hand, a lack of conflict can cause complacency and prevent creativity (Vecchio, 1991).

What should the supervisory participants do to resolve conflict? Most importantly, one must *respond*, not react. This means making an attempt to modify the expression of one's initial behavioral reaction. When confronted with a situation perceived as negative, one may at first feel angry. Depending on one's behavioral style, the expression of that emotion may need to be modified in order to keep the other participant from feeling rebellious or defensive. Typically, conflict resolution follows a pattern within the work arena:

1. Identify the problem.
   (I am assigned too many patients)

2. Determine if the conflict is important enough to act upon.
   (Quality of patient care is in jeopardy)

3. Establish a specific time and place to discuss the situation.
   (Ask for a meeting with supervisor)

4. Focus on observable problem behaviors.
   (I have a 10-patient caseload now, and the supervisor assigned three more this morning)

5. State your opinions but be open-minded to others.
   (I feel overwhelmed)

6. Determine the options available.
   (Group treatment, reassignment of patients, better time management, etc.)

7. Search the consequences of options.
   (Creative treatment method, overload on other staff, find information on time management, etc.)

8. Determine the best course of action.
   (Group treatment for patients with similar diagnoses)

9. Implement the course of action within an appropriate timeframe.

   (Develop group treatment protocol by Wednesday)

10. Evaluate the outcome and methods used.
    (Maintain outcome assessment on these patients for 1 month)

If given the opportunity to actively participate in the problem-solving process, most supervisees will perceive the supervisor as a caring person. The supervisee feels secure when the supervisor is aware and interested in employee problems.

How Much Supervision is Enough?

The amount of supervision can range from close supervision to minimal supervision. The OT profession has defined this as follows (AOTA, 1995); however, each profession generally has its own supervision requirements.

Close - requires daily, direct contact at the site of work.

Routine - requires direct contact at least every 2 weeks at the site of work with interim supervision occurring by other methods, such as by telephone or written communication.

General - requires at least monthly direct contact, with supervision available as needed by other methods.

Minimal - provided on an as needed basis and may be less than monthly.

This is only one attempt to define how much supervision a profession desires among its constituents. You will need to become familiar with any supervision guidelines developed for your particular profession.

The type of supervision required must be suitable to both the supervisor and the supervisee. The participants will need to make a commitment to re-evaluate the agreed upon amount and type of supervision at a predetermined time. Most supervisory situations allow for closer supervision as new participants are teamed into a new working relationship. Less supervision would be required as experienced clinicians are teamed together.

Management Styles

Historically, management styles have centered on three major types: authoritarian, democratic, and laissez-faire (Milkovich & Boudreau, 1991). The *authoritarian* leader typically makes decisions alone and tells others what to do, while the *democratic* leader involves others in the process of decision-making and allows a sense of shared responsibility. The *laissez-faire* leader tends to avoid decision-making and leaves it up to others. Although these styles remain stable, they are reminiscent of earlier thinking on the topic. Adaptation is a must if supervisory relationships are to grow in today's fast-paced world of work. A management style that is more diverse and supportive can address the needs of the present day workforce (Jameson and O'Mara, 1991).

Today's management team leader has adopted the role of *participative manager,* one who is proactive and facilitates others to reach objectives by allowing them to take part in the decision-making process (Shultz and Johnson, 1990). The needs of employees are considered in order to allow collaboration among workers instead of having competition between them. Collaboration allows for increased creativity, participation, commitment, and interdependence of the supervisory relationship. This leads to increased productivity, as well as job satisfaction and retention. A supervisory participant may or may not actually have control over the final decision to be made. The level of control each perceives that they have can have a global effect on both participants. Perceptions of how one can control events has an effect on self-esteem and confidence, in addition to one's physical and psychological well-being (Kagan and Evans, 1995). For example, if decisions are made only according to control issues (e.g., I'm the boss!), decision-making will be compromised. Without input from others, the *best* decision may not be made. However, if the supervisory relationship is one in which control is shared, dependent upon areas of expertise and trust, the relationship of those involved will thrive.

Novice to Master Supervision

The following tables illustrate four skill level combinations one might find at any time during his or her professional career. Each table defines what will need to happen in order to have an effective supervisory relationship. The tables also illustrate common blocks that might hinder the supervisory process.

The combinations include:

A. New Supervisor - New Supervisee (Table 11-3)
B. New Supervisor - Experienced Supervisee (Table 11-4)
C. Experienced Supervisor - New Supervisee (Table 11-5)
D. Experienced Supervisor - Experienced Supervisee (Table 11-6)

Conclusion

In today's health care market, changing roles demand the use of varied and comprehensive supervision practices. Effective supervision is one of the most difficult skills to master. This process needs to be *proactive* not *reactive.* It is a joint, not a solitary effort.

If practiced, the impact upon work relationships and professional development is immeasurable.

References

American heritage dictionary. (1976). New York, NY: Houghton Mifflin Company.

American Occupational Therapy Association (1995). Guide for supervision of occupational therapy personnel. *American Journal of Occupational Therapy, 49,* 1027-1028.

Buss, A., & Plomin, R. (1984). *Temperament: Early personality traits.* Hillsdale, NJ: Erlbaum.

Chess, S., & Thomas, A. (1986). *Temperament in clinical practice.* New York, NY: Guilford.

Jameson, D., & O'Mara, J. (1991). *Managing workforce 2000: Gaining the diversity advantage.* San Francisco, CA: Jossey-Bass.

Kagan, C., & Evans, J. (1995). *Professional interpersonal skills for nurses.* San Diego, CA: Singular Publishing Group, Inc.

Lerner, R. M., & Lerner, J. V. (1987). Children in their contexts: A goodness of fit model. In J. B. Lancaster, J. Altman, A. S. Rossi, & L. R. Sherrod, (Eds). *Parenting across the lifespan: Biosocial dimensions.* Chicago, IL: Aldine.

Levinson, H. (1962). Men, management and mental health. In T. Blechert, M. F. Christiansen, & N. Kari. Intraprofessional team building. *American Journal of Occupational Therapy, 41,* (9), 576-582.

Milkovich, G. T., & Boudreau, J. W. (1991). *Human resource management.* Boston, MA: Irwin, Inc.

Rothbart, M. K., & Derryberry, D. (1981). Development of individual differences in temperament. In M. E. Lamb, and A. L. Brown, (Eds). *Advances in Developmental Psychology, 1,* 37-86.

Schultz, R., & Johnson, A. C. (1990). *Management of hospitals and health services: Strategic issues and performance.* Baltimore, MD: C.V. Mosby.

Thomas, A., & Chess, S. (1977). *Temperament and development.* New York, NY: Brunner/Mazel.

TRANSACT, Inc. (1987) Liden, Dr. Craig B. *Clinical report.* Monroeville, PA.

Vecchio, R. P. (1991). *Organizational behavior.* Orlando, FL: The Dryden Press.

Table 11-3

NOVICE LEVEL - COMBINATION A: NEW SUPERVISOR - NEW SUPERVISEE

The Players:　　Supervisor: Beth, a Registered Occupational Therapist
　　　　　　　　Supervisee: Bob, a Certified Occupational Therapy Assistant

The Setting:　　Psychiatric Day Treatment Program

The Situation:　Both Bob and Beth are new graduates who were hired at approximately the same time. They are both traditional age students with limited life experience.

The Novice Supervisory Process	Supervisor Examples	Supervisee Examples
Flexibility Blocker: Don't have black and white thinking	Beth: "I was taught to do it the right way."	Bob: "I don't know enough to do that."
Flexibility: Do encourage risk-taking and accept the possibility of failure.	Beth: "I know you haven't done this before, so we'll go over it together."	Bob: "This will be a first for me, but I want to try."
Attitude Blocker: Don't have limited reflection and imagination.	Beth: "Why is he complaining, he makes good money."	Bob: "I work hard and all I ever hear is criticism."
Attitude: Do determine what motivates self and others (i.e., praise, money, power).	Beth: "What is important to you, Bob?"	Bob: "You're a great boss because you tell me what I need to know."
Trust Blocker: Don't let limited experience interfere.	Beth: "I need to make sure I know what is happening at all times."	Bob: "They didn't teach us that in school, I don't know where to look for that information."
Trust: Do maintain competence. Do show confidence in the work of others. Do explore the division of labor. DO find a mentor.	Beth: "Let's start with what skills you feel comfortable with."	Bob: "You've helped me learn so many new things. I believe you when you say I can do it."
Block to Respect: Don't have inaccurate assumptions of each other or self.	Beth: "I'm in charge, I'm the boss!"	Bob: "I'm just a COTA."
Respect: Do recognize each other as unique individuals.	Beth: "Don't underestimate your capabilities, I have a lot to learn too."	Bob: "I've gotten excellent training in my field."
Support Blocker: Don't fail to see the Big Picture.	Beth: "I already showed you how to do this once."	Bob: "We talked about doing it one way and now you are changing how to do it."
Support: Do reinforce the performance of others. Do view mistakes as a learning experience.	Beth: "We'll work on this until you you feel comfortable."	Bob: "Thanks for showing me how to do that technique. It helped me to understand the process."
Conflict Management Blocker: Don't fail to accept responsibility for your own actions.	Beth: "Because you can't follow directions, I have to talk to the doctor about this incident."	Bob: "That isn't the way you showed me."
Conflict Management: Do give and receive effective feedback.	Beth: "We reviewed all the note writing techniques. What was clear or not clear?"	Bob: "Let me summarize what we just discussed."

Table 11-4

INTERMEDIATE LEVEL - COMBINATION B: NEW SUPERVISOR - EXPERIENCED SUPERVISEE

The Players:	Supervisor: Chris, a Registered Nurse who is a new graduate Supervisee: Pat, a Certified Nurses Assistant
The Setting:	Helping Hands Skilled Nursing Facility
The Situation:	Pat has 20 years experience working in this facility.

The Intermediate Supervisory Process	Supervisor Examples	Supervisee Examples
Flexibility Blocker: Don't fail to participate in changed roles.	Chris: "In school they taught us that RN's were the ones responsible for taking vital signs."	Pat: "I always take my break at 10:15. I don't care what needs to be done."
Flexibility: Do accept that change occurs.	Chris: "I know that your break is very important to you. We can work around it."	Pat: "Let me explain to you what we have done in the past about that problem."
Attitude Blocker: Don't fail to listen openly.	Chris: "What can he tell me that I didn't already learn in school?"	Pat: "She's just a kid. What does she know?"
Attitude: Do cooperate and compromise in decision-making.	Chris: "That's different from the way I learned but I'm willing to try and see what works best for me."	Pat: "Chris, could you watch me build rapport with a patient and give me your feedback?"
Trust Blocker: Don't fail to self-disclose as appropriate to the work situation.	Chris: "If I tell Pat that I don't know the answer to that, he'll think that I don't know anything."	Pat: "It is important to talk to each patient for at least 5 minutes each day. Chris will think I'm just wasting time so I won't tell her."
Trust: Do be honest and sincere.	Chris: "Pat has a wealth of understanding of the unwritten rules here."	Pat: "Let me tell you about who you could talk to about that problem."
Respect Blocker: Don't fail to recognize life experience as contributing to effective relationships.	Chris: "Why can't he just retire!"	Pat: "She's just like all RN's! She'll never listen to me."
Respect: Do modify behavior in response to feedback that may differ from previous experience.	Chris: "Although it usually isn't done that way, Pat certainly has proved that he has the skills to do it."	Pat: "That's not how my old boss wanted me to do it, but the worst that can happen is that I'll learn something."
Support Blocker: Don't fail to set mutual goals.	Chris: "Nursing assistants have certain jobs to do and that's all they should do."	Pat: "Let Chris try to bathe three people at the same time! I never have time to talk with the patients."
Support: Do acknowledge a job well done. Do communicate your strengths and weaknesses.	Chris: "When I really look around, CNA's have skills I never really thought about!"	Pat: "Even though I've been here 20 years, I still need help with the computer system."
Conflict Management Blocker: Don't fail to have an open atmosphere for communication.	Chris: "I'll talk to you later if I get time."	Pat: "Chris is never around when I have questions."
Conflict Management: Do set regular meetings for feedback. Do maintain "open door" policy in verbal and non-verbal behaviors.	Chris: "We won't have time for our regular supervision meeting today, let's do it over lunch."	Pat: "I'll structure my questions so we can make the most of our supervisory meetings."

Table 11-5

INTERMEDIATE LEVEL - COMBINATION C: EXPERIENCED SUPERVISOR - NEW SUPERVISEE

The Players:	Supervisor: John, the Director of the Rehab Department Supervisee: Ted, a Licensed Physical Therapist who is a new graduate
The Setting:	Health Hospital
The Situation:	John is also a Licensed PT who has been in the position of Rehab Director for the past 5 years. Prior to working at Health Hospital, John was Rehab Director at another facility for 6 years.

The Intermediate Supervisory Process	Supervisor Examples	Supervisee Examples
Flexibility Blocker: Don't fail to understand one's response to change.	John: "Every time I want to make a policy change, you have to know the reason why."	Ted: "Things were running so smoothly, why do we have to do that?"
Flexibility: Do recognize that growth occurs through change.	John: "I see that since we changed the policy, you've been able to do the research you wanted."	Ted: "My confidence has grown since I keep that new supervisory log."
Attitude Blocker: Don't fail to encourage growth.	John: "Why is he complaining? When he developed that new treatment technique, I smiled and gave him a nod."	Ted: "If he really liked what I do, he'd tell me. Why should I ever try to advance?"
Attitude: Do understand that individual attitude expression varies according to the individual.	John: "I see you're frowning, what are your concerns?"	Ted: "When I frown, it usually means I don't understand."
Trust Blocker: Don't fail to participate in moving from a level of introductory learning to advanced learning.	John: "You did well during your probationary period. Just keep doing what you're doing!"	Ted: "This job is a piece of cake, I put in my hours and I'm outta here!"
Trust: Do be reliable and dedicated through an increasing level of competence.	John: "What new area would you like to master next?"	Ted: "What skill area can I work on next?"
Respect Blocker: Don't fail to accept the responsibility to look beyond the obvious.	John: "So, you're from the east end. It's amazing the determination those people have. I hope I can expect the same from you."	Ted: "He should know better, he was a PT before he became rehab director."
Respect: Do appreciate each other as individuals with varied cultures and histories.	John: "Tell me about yourself."	Ted: "What do you think your special skills are?"
Support Blocker: Don't fail to offer feedback in a constructive and positive way.	John: "That was a good job!"	Ted: "What does he mean good job? I guess that means there's nothing else I need to do."
Support: Do encourage others.	John: "We reviewed what you need to do, how to do it, and a target date. Any questions?"	Ted: "If we figure this out together, I'll have more time to do what is most important."
Conflict Management Blocker: Don't fail to focus on observable behaviors.	John: "No wonder Ted can't get his work done. He just doesn't think."	Ted: "Let John worry about how to solve my patient overload problem. It's his job."
Conflict Management: Do actively participate in the problem-solving process.	John: "If we work on this together, everyone will benefit."	Ted:"Thanks for helping me brainstorm to think of ways to solve the patient overload."

Table 11-6

EXPERT LEVEL - COMBINATION D: EXPERIENCED SUPERVISOR - EXPERIENCED SUPERVISEE

The Players: Supervisor: Annette, Chief Executive Officer
Supervisee: Jane, Vice President

The Setting: Allied Health Group, contract company

The Situation: Annette has 20 years experience in health care and business. Jane has 15 years experience in health care. They were both hired by the company at the same time.

The Expert Supervisory Process	Supervisor Examples	Supervisee Examples
Flexibility Blocker: Don't fail to look at all options and choices.	Annette: "Even though you have experience, since my background is in business, I should make all business decisions."	Jane: "Well, I guess that's the end of that!"
Flexibility: Do match the best person to the job.	Annette: "I see that your experience more than qualifies you for this task. What help do you need?"	Jane: "Did you know that I was responsible for a 1 million dollar budget at my last job?"
Attitude Blocker: Don't fail to modify your own attitude.	Annette: "Sometimes Jane is just too persistent."	Jane: "Sometimes Annette isn't realistic."
Attitude: Do understand that strengths and weaknesses are relative to the individual and the situation.	Annette: "Jane's persistence will help balance my procrastination."	Jane: "Sometimes I need someone to help me stop and think things through."
Trust Blocker: Don't fail to be sincere.	Annette: "Jot down your ideas for the company's new 5-year strategic plan and I'll decide if they fit with my vision."	Jane: "Jot down! Does she really want my ideas if she already has her vision?"
Trust: Do develop shared expectations through communication and compromise.	Annette: "There are a few expectations that are not negotiable, like integrity, etc. Everything else is open for discussion."	Jane: "If my ideas aren't used this time, there's always next time!"
Respect Blocker: Don't fail to accurately assess behaviors by neglecting to communicate.	Annette: "Jane hates new duties assigned on short notice, so I'll give this task to someone else."	Jane: "Why didn't she ask me to do that? She should trust me by now."
Respect: Do recognize how behavioral traits impact the supervisory process.	Annette: "Jane, I know you hate last minute assignments but you're the only one I trust for this. How can I help you?"	Jane: "I'm glad you asked, I would like to delegate the last portion to Sam, he's the expert in that area."
Support Blocker: Don't fail to offer support when difficult decisions need to be made.	Annette: "I delegated that decision to Jane. Let me go talk to her and we'll change it."	Jane: "Annette had to make a tough decision. Of course, it's not what I would have done."
Support: Do be loyal.	Annette: "Jane, it was the right decision. I'm behind you."	Jane: "I've walked in Annette's shoes. Those decisions aren't easy."
Conflict Management Blocker: Don't fail to relinquish control when necessary.	Annette: "Look Jane you're a good VP, but if I let you do that then everybody would want to."	Jane: "I can't wait until the shareholders find out about this!"
Conflict Management: Do mutually decide on the importance of the issue.	Annette: "Jane, what do you think is the best or worst that will happen in this situation?"	Jane: "Have you thought about what the shareholders might do?"

Exercises for Supervisory Process

Believe It or Not

Goal: To illustrate the differences in individual attitudes and behaviors.

Participants: Small group of 6 to 12 participants seated in a circle.

Materials: Flipchart, pen, soft foam ball (or other soft object)

Procedure:

1. Write the following statements on the flip chart (1 per page).
   - Supervisors should always:
   - Supervisees should always:
   - If supervisors want to solve problems he or she should always:
   - If supervisees want to solve problems he or she should always:
   - When a supervisor disagrees, he or she should always:
   - When a supervisee disagrees, he or she should always:

2. The facilitator reads the first topic sentence, and then throws the ball to someone in the group.

3. The catcher reads the topic sentence, fills in the blank with his or her belief, and then tosses the ball to someone else in the group.

4. The process continues until a variety of responses are made to the first topic sentence. Then move on in turn to the other sentences.

5. Point out that each sentence contains the word "should". Try the same activity with the word should eliminated. You will find that responses will change.

Discussion Questions

1. What did you learn about the attitudes or beliefs of other people?

2. How similar or different are they?

3. What happens when we expect others to behave in a certain way and they act differentially?

4. Point out that each sentence includes the absolute qualifier "always." How are our attitudes affected when we think in terms of always, every, all, etc.?

5. How do we develop these attitudes?

6. How can we prevent these attitudes from occurring?

Additional Resources

Bair, J. & Gray, M. (1985). *The occupational therapy manager.* Baltimore, MD: American Occupational Therapy Association.

Drafke, M. W. (1994). *Working in healthcare: What you need to know to succeed.* Philadelphia, PA: F.A. Davis.

Early, M. B. (1996). *Mental health concepts and techniques for the occupational therapy assistant.* Philadelphia, PA: Lippincott-Raven.

Littauer, F. (1983). *How to understand others by understanding yourself: Personality plus.* Old Tappan, NJ: Fleming H. Revell Company.

Purtilo, R., & Haddad, A. (1996). *Health professional and patient interaction.* Philadelphia, PA: W.B. Saunders Company.

Navarra, T., Lipkowitz, M. A., & Navarra, J.A., Jr. (1990). *Therapeutic communication: A guide to effective interpersonal skills for health care professionals.* Thorofare, NJ: SLACK Incorporated.

Chapter Twelve

Verbal Communication

Evelyn Anne Mocek, OTR/L, CHT

E. Nelson Clark, MS, OTR/L

Picture the following:

Two men walking in opposite directions:

Man one: "Hi Bob, how are you doing?"

Man two: "Just fine Jim, how about yourself?"

A doctor and patient:

Doctor: "So what brings you here today?"

Patient: "Well doctor, I have this pain in my left shoulder when I lift up my arm and cough."

Doctor: "Does your arm hurt any other time?"

Patient: "No, just when I do that."

Doctor: "Then don't do it."

Human Resources representative and prospective employee for a grocery packer:

Representative: "So what strengths do you feel you have that would make you a good grocery packer?"

Employee: "Well, I am an upbeat individual, who has a strong sense of order."

Verbal communication encompasses every aspect of one's life. This is seen in the cooing and echoing of an infant, to the professional communication in the business arena, as well as interpersonal relationships with other persons.

Verbal Communication Defined

There is no single dictionary definition of the term *verbal communication*. Separate definitions of the component words are as follows:

Verbal: 1) of relating to, or associated with words; 2) concerned with words only, rather than with content or ideas (*American Heritage*, 1992). Concerned with or using words for effect rather than meaning (*Webster's*, 1981).

Communication: 1) the exchange of thoughts, messages, or information as by speech, signals, writing or behavior; 2) the art and technique of using words effectively and with grace in imparting ones ideas (*American Heritage*, 1992). The act or action of imparting or transmitting facts or information (Gove, 1981).

The working definition of the term *verbal communication* as used in this chapter is the act of speaking words both for their effect and meaning when transmitting information and/or ideas to another individual.

Model of Communication

The process of communication is an ongoing, never static and never-ending task. It's perhaps the most important skill one has.

A baseline model for *all* communication is as follows: (Casmir, 1974):

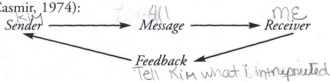

$Sender \longrightarrow Message \longrightarrow Receiver$

$Feedback$

The process for communication following the above model is: a message is sent, and the eyes and ears of the receiver take in the message. Then the receiver encodes the message using his or her own process of sorting and selecting information. Finally, the receiver provides feedback. Note that this is a continuous process, not a static line going one way. An example of static verbal communication is talking to an individual who is comatose. The sender is talking to the patient (receiver); however, there is no feedback as to whether the message is heard or understood.

An exercise demonstrating how verbal communication can break down follows:

- Objective
  - Use the childhood game of telephone to demonstrate how a receiver may not be getting the message accurately from the sender.
- Instructions
  - Have small group of people (preferably 6 to 12), arranged in a line or circle.
  - The sender must whisper the message to the receiver next to him or her.
  - Only *one* attempt at sending the message is allowed.
  - Receiver then sends the message to the next individual.
  - Last receiver provides feedback by stating the message out loud to the group.
- Message
  - Any tongue twister can be used for message.
  - If possible, make up tongue twisters so familiarity will not play a factor in message reception.
  - Sample message:
    "Harry the health care houdini helps Henderson hobble happily homeward".

Factors Affecting Communication

Personal Style

All individuals have a personal style of communicating, i.e., some people talk with their hands emphasizing their points, while others may have a tremor in their voice when discussing emotional issues. External environmental factors can influence one's style. Regional accents and speed of delivery are good examples of environmental factors. This is illustrated by an individual who may have grown up in the southern United States, where the speed of delivery and accents are slow and deliberate. If that individual moved to New York City, he or she may have a difficult time adjusting to the fast, abrupt style of speech that is common there.

Inherent Qualities

Inherent qualities within each individual's communication style are equally important. Examples of this include inflection and tonal quality. A person who has a deep voice, such as the well known actor and announcer James Earl Jones, may instill confidence and comfort as compared to television actress Fran Dresher's nasal tones. Inherent qualities may also be related to the specifics of the language spoken. Case in point: the French and Spanish languages use a gender based style of communication. Additionally, education and/or social class may be inherent in the communication style. In England, there is a class distinction made between cockney and other Londoners due to the specific style and colloquialisms inherent with the cockney style. The play *My Fair Lady* illustrates this point.

Quality of communication style exists within all languages; however, it is more concerned with *how* one says what is said. If an individual controls the communication style, he or she can control the outcome of most interactions, such as using indirectness or politely refusing to answer questions, versus loud shouting. With pig latin for example, individuals using this style can effectively limit information passed only to others who understand the meanings of the words. The conversations that one both listens to and partakes in shapes his or her personal worlds. An excellent example of this is seen within the television show Frasier. Dr. Crane tends to use a very highbrow, intellectual, and affected style when communicating with his brother and a more generic, comfortable speaking style with his father.

Communication Basics

Language operates on two basic levels. *Denotative* language is the literal meaning of a word, i.e., cat is a cat. *Connotative* language is the meaning of a word through a process of association, i.e., she is such a cat (Beebe & Beebe, 1991). Because of these two interrelated processes of language, we must be aware of hidden meanings in the words we choose during verbal communication that could skew our intended message. An example of how the meaning of a word can change is the word "gay". Originally the word meant to be happy, relating to a celebration (*American Heritage*, 1992). However in today's society, it is now generally related to an individual who participates in a homosexual or lesbian relationship. "He was a gay man" in the 1940's would mean he was happy, but now has an entirely different meaning. Geographical location can also skew the meaning of a word. For example, within western Pennsylvania/Pennsylvania Dutch areas, "We need to red up the room" does not mean paint the room red, but to clean the room.

Power of Communication

Communication is very powerful. Words create one's world. They color an individual's perception and reality. A well-timed word or phrase can override sensory perception. A good example of this is as follows: A professor brought cookies to class. After the students tasted and appreciated the flavor, he informed the class that the recipe included crushed dog biscuits. The students promptly spit out any cookies in their mouths and had a dramatic change in the perception of the cookie's taste. Subsequently the professor did reveal that the cookies were baked with normal ingredients. (Beebe & Beebe, 1991).

This example demonstrates that even though the taste buds were communicating that the cookies were excellent, the revelation that dog biscuits were used "colored" the sensory perceptions. These perceptions are made based on many things. Past experiences play a role; perhaps we tried dog biscuits as a child. Our values also contribute to the perception of taste. Most individuals feel that dog food is substandard for human consumption. Also involved is an inherent protective response from possible poison. Many children use nebulous perceptions to make decisions regarding food choices, for example, tater tots vs. french fries. If tater tots are presented as something new, the child may refuse to try them; however, if they are told that tater tots are round french fries, a positive reaction may result.

How Do We Communicate?

Pitch and Intonation

Verbal communication is not done in isolation. When communicating to another human being or creature, intonation, body language, and pitch are also used to effectively make a point. The necessity of tonal changes (pitch) cannot be understated. Imagine telling a puppy chewing on your new shoes, "No", in a low monotone.

How effective would it be? Or when talking to an 80-year-old individual with a hearing loss who refuses to wear his or her hearing aid. If the pitch is high, it is difficult to hear. The individual will probably hear one word in four. You could be saying, "Hi, how are you doing today?" The person hears the words *Hi* and *doing*, and responds with "Nothing", assuming that you asked "What are you doing?" This interchange demonstrates how quickly verbal communication can break down. The best example of intonation and pitch playing a strong role is the telephone. Communication via the phone is based solely on verbal communication, as there is no face to face contact between the speakers. What is said and how it is said, reflect on how the message is received. At one time or another every individual has developed an impression of someone via the phone by the primary context of their tone, e.g., operators perceived as friendly or unfriendly, and acquaintances perceived as feeling upbeat or down.

Living in the 20th and progressing to the 21st century, one is constantly bombarded with information that is both positive and negative. Television and the Internet are becoming much more interactive, thus allowing for more direct, real-time, video/verbal interaction versus written/pictorial communication. A good example of how the television is used for combined verbal/pictorial communication is with children's toys. The timing of the commercials are always during prime child viewing, and the tone of voice used to promote the product is geared to inspire excitement for the product. Other techniques are the body language of the actors and the types of print on the products' packaging indicating fun. Conversely, negative information is generally imparted in a solemn voice with little or no facial expression, exemplified in the evening news or when there is a major breaking news story. The best example of this is the terrorist attack on the Oklahoma City Federal Building. The announcers all had flat tonal expression in their voices when the news story broke, and after the pictures of the individuals injured and killed were shown, especially the children, the tone and pitch changed as emotions surfaced.

Intelligence and Prejudice

When a message is communicated, information about the individual communicating is also subtly provided, including one's educational level and any inherent prejudices. An individual stating that, "Only the people who graduate from an Ivy league school and winter on the

French Riviera are fit to associate with," would convey certain messages. Other information, such as do we believe in what we are saying or is this a pleasant or unpleasant task, is also imparted. Even the words chosen relay information about an individual. A 5-year-old using the word antidisestablishmentarianism in context and appropriately in a sentence would be considered very intelligent. When a professional speaker uses the same word, it is not unexpected of that person and therefore intelligence is not judged to be particularly high.

Communication of Values

Ideally speaking, there is a common value system expected within those with whom one communicates. These include:

- Interest - maintaining eye contact and responding with appropriate questions.
- Dedication - following through with what is discussed.
- Skill - handles self like a professional.
- Ability - able to communicate the why and wherefore.
- Truth - lets the chips fall where they may.
- Sensitivity - cares about others' feelings.
- Honesty - can be trusted.
- Sincerity - sounds like they really mean what they say.

Sincerity is the one, almost fundamental factor in verbal communication (Casmir, 1974). All of us have experienced casual interpersonal contacts when no values are expected to be demonstrated or any information provided. A standard example is when one walks past another person and asks "How are you?"

As one grows, verbal communication skills develop by leaps and bounds. Patterns of consistent behavior are always looked for in what is said, i.e., sincerity. The baseline experiences used to evaluate the message or the ability to send the correct message also develops as one grows. An example of this is when a child is learning the difference between lying and making a promise. Many children hear from their parents, "we'll see" or "maybe," when a request is made. When this response is received, the outcome is unknown. However, "I promise," is considered to be a definite. If the promise is not kept, the child may perceive that the adult "lied" to them. A natural urge to judge, evaluate, and approve (disapprove) another person's statement occurs in all communication. This is a *learned* skill versus an *inherent* skill. This is represented in the statement, "Santa Claus lives at the North Pole." A child

will accept this statement as fact, as they generally do not evaluate what is communicated. An adult will look for proof or indications of a falsehood via how the statement was made and the body language used during the statement, e.g., eyes lowered indicating lying.

Types of Communication

Family

Verbal communication skills are first evident within the family. This is the primary group that shapes our communication style and self-image. Dyadic communication (one to one) is the most frequent kind of human contact. A child must learn to successfully interpret another person's communication and in turn respond in an appropriate, understandable manner. Initially, the infant learns that crying illicits a response. The caretaker will see to the baby's immediate needs, i.e., food, changing diapers, or general handling and cuddling. Later, the child may smile to prolong a contact or babble to attract attention, and might illicit a positive non-verbal reaction from the parent, i.e., a smile. This encourages repetition of the behavior that got the smile from the caregivers. In this manner, the child effectively engages in a two-way conversation. As development progresses, the baby imitates adult sounds, facial expressions, and symbolic speech (gestures), engages the caregiver, and contributes to the amount and quality of attention received. If a baby is passive and silent, the parent has no auditory or visual feedback to gauge the interaction with the child. A good example of this is autistic children. Spontaneous speech is critical for social interactions as well as requesting and obtaining material goods, information, and attention (Gains & Halpern-Felsher, 1995). As a child grows, he or she demonstrate an ever-expanding array of sounds and words to express his or her mood and needs. He or she generally starts learning family names, important objects (food, drink, etc.), and toys or play things used in his or her environment. Continuing to grow, interactive play with both the family and other children requires a more comprehensive verbal repertoire, organization of what is communicated, as well as cooperation (LeCroy, 1983). Also within any family are intimate communications. These communications impart personal information and caring, i.e., "I love you". This is the most revealing and personally satisfying type of communication. This allows for observations and feedback without distortions caused by the environment. This intimate dyadic communication is dependent on trust. It is also a major source of miscommunication. Many plays and entertainment shows are based on this miscommunication, e.g., *Taming of the Shrew* and *Midsummer's Night Dream,* and contemporary shows such as *Home Improvement* and *When Harry Met Sally.*

Others Outside the Family Unit

As individuals grow, they progress from contact with just the family unit to include other individuals and later groups via school. Children bring the unique family communication styles to the groups encountered in school. They then hopefully find a common ground between what is the norm for home and the norm in a group. An example of this is a boy who has been encouraged to discuss how parental actions affected his feelings at home (hurt feelings when yelled at). When the child uses the same technique within a group of his peers, he may be told that he is a sissy. The desire to fit in with the group results in less acknowledgment of how an individual's actions affect the child's feelings and more stoic "manly" expressions used. Interpersonal skills describe the ability to effectively interact with a variety of people, as well as communicate an individual's wants and needs. Styles that have proven effective before tend to be used. Typical styles used are directness when assistance is needed ("Could you help me"), or whining to achieve results ("But you never told me, and I can't").

Group Communication Skills

ROLES

When we start school we begin to move from primarily interpersonal dyadic communication, to group communications. Within group communication, we all have roles we assume. Roles that might emerge in the early years include:

1. *Information Seekers* - these individuals are not afraid to ask questions.

2. *Information Gatherers* - these individuals are not afraid to speak their minds; confident.

3. *Coordinators/Leaders* - these individuals are very open, give ideas to follow.

4. *Encouragers* - these individuals are free to give praise to others.

5. *Followers* - these individuals are the ones who listen well and follow directions well.

6. *Aggressors* - these individuals may want to join in; however, they tend to interrupt and take the ball, rather than ask "Can I play?"

7. *Recognition Seekers* - these individuals may either be the class clown making jokes of unmet needs, or may diminish the importance by saying "that's dumb".

8. *Withdrawn* - these individuals do not participate or voice needs.

Imagine any playground or group of children playing. Each of the above roles can be seen within that group of children. Of note, the roles are not static. A child can at one moment be a leader, and then change to a follower, allowing someone else to lead.

In the typically large classroom, strict guidelines for behaviors are generally established; however, when the class breaks into small groups, the individual must learn the skill of when to speak, when to listen, and when to interrupt or not interrupt. Consider the example of a child who has not learned this skill. When the caretaker is on the phone or talking with other adults, the child will repeatedly interrupt without any regard for the others in the group.

Small group communication allows for, and expects, contributions from each individual in the group. This is accomplished by utilizing information based on each individual's background, experiences, and feelings. These groups incorporate skills learned earlier in life and previously described roles emerge. Within the work environment, we are generally assigned to groups with limited control of membership or choice of others in the group.

Group Process

Communication has two distinct group processes: the *Learning Group* and the *Problem-Solving Group.* The major distinction between the two is that with the problem-solving group, there is a distinct task to be accomplished, usually within a set timeframe. Examples of problem-solving groups are search committees for employees and fact-finding committees. A learning group allows for members to form their own decisions from the information gained during the process. Typical examples of learning groups are literary, political, or religious discussions. The vital aspect of both types of groups is that all members are involved, interact, and communicate with each other. The maximum size for groups, where *all* are expected to actively participate, tends to be nine members. Small groups are frequently a fact of life. Think of the number of groups (e.g., charitable, religious, political) we participate in daily.

Practical Application of Verbal Communication Skills

Interviews versus Social Interactions

When one enters the work environment, typically one of the most stressful, yet necessary, types of verbal communication is the interview. Frequently this skill is used to determine if an individual fits a position or task. Generally this is an example of a problem-solving group. Two distinct yet related types of interviews are utilized in this process. *Information-seeking* interviews are the typical job interview. Generally, the interviewer asks specific questions and the interviewee responds to each question. This type of interview seeks to determine if the interviewee's specific skills and personal style fit the needs required by the person doing the interview. *Problem-solving* interviews are generally more difficult. This type of interview involves intense feelings or difficult issues, i.e., reprimanding or praising an employee. In this type of interview, one seeks to determine the cause of a problem, underlying factors, hidden agendas, and possible solutions. This may be illustrated by a problem employee who repeatedly comes to work late. The first difficult communication skill is the actual confrontation of the issue with the individual involved. Then, following determination of cause, effect, and frequency (through dyadic discussion), a solution is reached. This type of interview requires a strong ability to communicate succinctly and effectively on a one to one basis. While emotions may run strongly, they cannot interfere with the interview or the solution process.

The primary difference between interviews and social dyadic conversations is that interviews require preplanning and are more structured. The participants plan what to say and the interviewers determine what questions need to be asked. Social conversations, on the other hand, generally are spontaneous. There are, however, specific unwritten (or unspoken) guidelines that are followed. These include the exclusion of topics such as politics, religion, and personal trials and tribulations in a given situation. These guidelines can follow cultural/social or gender based perspectives.

Feedback

When individuals are progressing within a desired profession, they tend to move along a continuum. The starting point is one of insecurity, where few questions are asked of direct supervisors. Individuals tend to expect one-way communication. They expect to be literally told what to do and how to do it. Employees generally do not feel either empowered enough to question a direct supervisor, or they do not have the skills required to provide "qualified" input to a situation. As skills improve, a sense of greater security is evidenced by the increased feedback experienced between the individuals and supervisors. Most supervisors expect subordinates to take the initiative and be responsible for asking questions, and seeing that their individual needs are met. This requires a baseline communication skill that inspires confidence, as well as the willingness to take risks during dyadic communications.

Effective feedback is therefore an important verbal communication component. Referring to the basic process of communication, feedback is required within the circle of the communication to maintain the integrity as well as momentum of the process. Being able to give, as well as receive, feedback is imperative to good communication. Providing feedback requires certain baseline factors that maintain its effectiveness. These include:

Be Specific! Without specifics, the receiver is unable to appropriately respond to the satisfaction of the sender. A good example of this is the typical parent/child relationship. When the parent says, "Because I said so, that's why!", what response is expected of the child? There has been no clarification to specifically *why*, just generalities. As we grow, another broadbased statement that is frequently heard is "Everyone else does it." The general response of the receiver is: Who is everyone? Within the work environment, one of the most frustrating examples of generalities is "Other duties as indicated." No specific tasks are assigned, therefore allowing for a very broad-based interpretation.

Timeliness. When providing feedback, the more immediate the response, the better. Granted, this is not always possible, especially if further data is required; however, procrastination is not indicated. Timeliness frequently falls to the wayside, especially when the feedback is difficult or painful. Poor feedback timeliness is frequently seen in the work environment, e.g.:

When requesting a day off, John talked to his supervisor Bill. Bill told John he would let him know. It has now been 2 weeks since John talked to Bill, and the day he wanted off to see his son graduate pre-school is tomorrow. John is frustrated and angry with Bill because he can't tell his son he will be there.

"I" messages. Defensiveness is a frequent response when receiving feedback. "I" messages help to alleviate this natural tendency. Feedback can sometimes be misunderstood as a personal attack upon one's skills or personality. Most children start early with using "I" messages. Children perceive how hurtful it is to their parent when they say, "I hate you!" Of course this is just a way of venting; however, within verbal communication, it is an early attempt at owning and transmitting feelings. As one grows into adulthood, "I" messages are used to aid in correcting behavior, and changing perceptions. An example using an "I" message is as follows:

When you told the doctor that we couldn't provide for his orders, I felt that you were not confident with my skills while you were on vacation.

The "I" message allowed for the sender to express feelings, while also giving specifics as to what occurred to cause those feelings. Contrast the above "I" message with the statement, "You never trust me." Note that the three basic fundamentals discussed (specifics, timeliness, and "I" messages) are *not* present in this broadbased statement.

Perception. Another important component of effective feedback is understanding how the receiver perceives events and the resulting reactions. A case in point is seen in the following:

John is talking to the secretary. His boss, Paula, comes in and asks for assistance with a patient. Paula may perceive the interaction on the basic information relayed - I need help. John, on the other hand, may be feeling that he was neglecting the patient while talking to the secretary about a movie seen last night, and that Paula made the request to make him feel guilty. In fact, Paula was not asking for the help to make John feel that he was not doing his job.

This "getting to know" the other person also includes reflecting on one's own personal history, and how that affects an individual's standards and actions. How each individual acts or responds is based on past learning experiences, and whether that action was successful or not. If a child learns that whining will get him the toy he desires, feedback to the contrary may not be effective. Consistency is key when providing feedback. Using the above example, if the same message of requesting help is used in other situations, John may realize that Paula is only asking for help, and the perceived negative slant to the feedback is negated.

Openness. The last component within the feedback process is the need to remain open to each other's ideas, skills, and work performance. If one assumes that he or she has all the answers, or insists on giving all the answers, that individual may miss valuable feedback, for example:

Tom is a therapist who specializes in working with hand injured patients. Larry has an injury requiring that his hand manipulation skills be improved. Tom has a standard set of exercises for this task. If he doesn't listen to Larry, he will not benefit from Larry's ideas about a technique that he used to improve his manipulation skills when he was studying to be a musician. Openness to the feedback during this process allowed Tom to grow and gain a new and perhaps better exercise approach for possible use with his other patients.

Health Care Communication

Medical Jargon

Verbal communication in a profession has its own special needs. Almost all professions have their own "language". A good example of this is medical jargon. An individual who works within the health care environment as a professional tends to speak on a level generally not understood by a lay person. A sample of this medical jargon is as follows: "The patient has had a massive intercranial contusion resulting in hemiparesis", versus "The person had a bad bump on the head causing the one side of his body to be weak."

Effective verbal communication within the health care environment is imperative. Health care professionals communicate with patients, families, other professionals, and the general public on a daily basis.

Communication with Patients

Direct communication with a patient is generally considered to be one of the most important but sometimes least-used approaches. A typical example is when the doctor may only talk to parents, and neglect to ask the child questions that may impact on treatment decisions. Without this mutual communication, the parent and/or child may not perceive themselves as a viable partner in the decision-making process.

Verbal communication has been found to be one of the key components to effectively treating and providing care to all ages. Fowkes (1988) introduced an approach that uses the acronym LEARN:

        L = listen (to the patient's concerns)
        E = explain (what is to occur)
        A = acknowledge (fears)
        R = recommend (further treatment)
        N = negotiate (as needed)

This approach can be utilized as an effective tool across any continuum, age, or culture. Equally important in any therapeutic communication is non-verbal communication. This includes a gentle touch (if socially acceptable), eye contact with the patient when talking to him or her, and the tone of voice.

Communication with Other Professionals

The quality of work done by an individual is directly impacted by the way he or she communicates. Therefore, the quality of communication may affect the professional status of that individual. It is expected that when communication regarding a patient's progress is documented, a thorough, but brief, description of the treatment is made to the medical team. Imagine a progress note summary that simply states: " Mr. Jones did good in therapy today". The receiver of this message will make judgments regarding the sender. The other extreme is a report that is excessive, rambling, and in general too time-consuming to understand. Time is an important commodity in health care.

How the health care provided is communicated to third party payers, such as insurance companies and government agencies, directly affects monetary reimbursement. Communication in the medical profession might be compared to the sales profession. Within sales, the objective is to convince an individual to purchase a product. In medicine, the objective is to provide treatment alternatives that will allow complete care in the briefest amount of time. Communication in this sense is a combination of sales and medical objectives. The need for services, plus the sales aspect in convincing the payer to pay for services, are equally important when communicating a message.

Educational Communication

Health care professionals also provide educational opportunities for patients, staff, and the community. This is done via inservices and networking. Inservices are generally formalized presentations on a specific topic to assembled professionals or lay persons. When providing or participating in an inservice, the message that is being conveyed is done in such a manner as to resemble academic teaching.

Networking provides for established relationships with other professionals and agencies. It also allows contacts for information, advice, and professional support. Networking is generally very open and spontaneous (this resembles the didactic style of communication between friends).

Other Aspects of Verbal Communication in Health Care

Verbal interactions do affect other areas of patient care. The saying, "the squeaky wheel gets the grease," often applies to the care the professional renders to the client. When a client is viewed as a constant complainer, the care can be negatively affected. However, unless an individual speaks up and makes his or her needs known, the health care professional is often left to his or her own assumptions and evaluations. Quite often health care providers have been misled by subjective complaints from the patient, only to find another cause for the illness or ailment. In this area of verbal interactions, health care professionals must be keenly aware of vocal inflections, on both their parts and the clients'. This allows for a more objective transmission of accurate information, and thereby provision of appropriate care and support.

Verbal interaction within health care will often transmit other values including caring and concern for the well-being of the patient. If the professional is to communicate the value of caring and the sincerity of his or her efforts, then the professional must be dedicated to these beliefs to the point of sounding sincere. One only has to listen to political rhetoric to examine this idea. Can a good salesman sell something he or she does not endorse? On a bad day, can a health care worker communicate caring and concern to the patient, while preoccupied with personal concerns? The authors tend to believe that an individual *can* convey certain messages while feeling the opposite. However, this a skill that requires practice and awareness.

Developing Verbal Communication Awareness

While the previous topics are designed to encourage thought and dialogue, one must now gain awareness of how verbal communication in differing circumstances affects professional behavior. The first stage of developing an awareness of how one communicates is to simply ask coworkers or peers. A useful approach might be to say, "I need to know how I affect you when I talk to you. I am concerned about whether my voice communicates my ideas and observations accurately and honestly. Please give me your honest opinion. How do I sound to you?" If direct dialogue is not one's style, perhaps a checklist of behaviors can be given to an evaluator. Determining communication awareness involves a personal risk; however, it is an important step.

Developing an awareness leading to change is often a scary path. After gaining from the objective observations of others regarding one's personal communication style, the next step will be to address areas of weakness. Role playing with professional peers will allow experimentation and feedback. The following is a suggestion for a clinical or classroom inservice in verbal communications.

- Objective
  - Communicate in such a manner that it would influence the listener into believing the severity of the incident by the way it was communicated
  - Fabricate several clinical incidents and attempt to give them differing meanings by the way that they are communicated.
- Instructions
  - The communication can only state facts
  - The listener must objectively attempt to extract the correct data
  - Attempt to communicate in various ways
    - Humorously
    - With anger
    - Matter-of-factly
    - Overly-concerned
- Situation
  - The patient fell while transferring from bed to chair
  - You were not watching at the time
  - The patient laughed at first
  - The patient later complained of a painful wrist
  - Listener to remain objective and attempt to extract objective data

In the above exercise, the *way* that an individual describes facts or data should illustrate that the actual events or outcomes can be affected. If an individual transmits the facts humorously, he or she may not be presenting the information in an appropriately concerned or serious method. This could result in delayed or even lack of care for the patient. Conversely, some individuals are doomsayers, and transmit information in a negative manner. This could result in over attention or unnecessary procedures for the patient. One can readily see the inherent danger in both of these styles. Other illustrations of this point include: the client who laughs off serious pain to cover up an illness; an aide who describes a serious incident in a humorous manner to disguise neglect; or a co-worker who attempts to gain status or attention by making a situation more serious than is necessary. Again, by making these individuals aware of how they are communicating, or by clarifying the message transmitted, time and money in the provision of health care could be saved.

Listening

One cannot speak of the development of verbal communication without discussing briefly the skill of listening. You hear over 1 billion words a year. However, hearing and listening are not the same. Hearing is a physiological process, whereas listening is the process of selecting, attending, understanding, and remembering. *Selecting* and *attending* are interrelated, allowing one to focus on specific sounds and information; for example, a mother's ability to hear her child within a group of children. *Understanding* assigns meaning to the information, and *remembering* incorporates the message into memory.

Effective listening as a skill is rarely used. Barriers to effective listening include:

- Prematurely rejecting a topic
- Information overload
- Preoccupation with personal concerns
- Attending to outside distractions
- Judging the message too quickly
- Communication style of speaker

To be an effective listener one should look for nonverbal cues to the message, control personal emotions, focus on the speaker, listen before making judgments, mentally summarize the key points, listen for major ideas, and attempt to adapt to the speaker's style of communication (Beebe & Beebe, 1991).

In summary, verbal communication requires practicing sending a message, evaluation of feedback provided by the receiver, and still more practice. As the saying goes, practice makes perfect.

References

Beebe, S. A., & Beebe, S. J. (1991). *Public speaking: An audience centered approach.* Englewood Cliffs, NJ: Prentice Hall.

Casmir, F. L. (1974). *Interaction: An introduction to speech communication.* Columbus, OH: Charles E. Merrill Publishing Co.

Gains, R., & Halpern-Felsher, B. L. (1995). Language preference and communication development of a hearing and deaf twin pair. *American Annal of the Deaf, 140 (1),* 47-55.

Gove, P. B. (Ed.) (1981). *Webster's third new international dictionary unabridged.* Springfield, MA: G & C Merrian Company.

Houghton Mifflin (1992). *The American heritage dictionary of the English language.* 3rd edition. New York, NY: Houghton Mifflin Company.

Howe, M. C., & Schwartzberg, S. L. (1995). *A functional approach to group work in occupational therapy.* 2nd edition. Philadelphia, PA: J. B. Lippincott.

LeCroy, C. W. (1983). *Social skills training for children and youth.* New York, NY: Haworth Press.

Llorens, L. (1993). Ethnogeriatrics: Implications for occupational and physical therapy. *Physical and Occupational Therapy in Geriatrics, 11(3),* 59-67.

Exercise for Verbal Communication

- Objectives:
    - Provide opportunity to use communication skills
    - Use interviewing techniques
    - Use feedback techniques
    - Provide opportunity to explore how communication cycle is continuous

- Instructions:
    - Each individual involved will be assigned a historical figure
    - Could be done either with only the individual knowing who they are supposed top be, or only the individual NOT knowing who they are (name attached to back)
    - Initially, questions can be basic and answered with yes/no or very short answer
        - Samples:
            - Male versus female   - Occupation
            - Living versus dead   - Time period lived
    - Following this initial information gathering period, more in-depth questions can be asked regarding character, accomplishments, strengths, weaknesses
    - Interviewee may ask for information from more that one player to aid in information gathering potential

- Sample historical figures:

Female	Male
- Marie Antoinette	- Henry the Eighth
- Amelia Earhart	- William Shakespeare
- Louisa May Alcott	- Albert Einstein
- Mother Theresa	- Desmond Tutu
- Queen Victoria	- Dr. Martin Luther King
- Eleanor Roosevelt	- Jesse James
- Joan of Arc	- Moses

- Follow-up:
    - Review process of interviewing - What was effective/ineffective? How were character issues regarding historical person ascertained through the interview?
    - Review process of listening - What information was missed? What barriers were noted during the interviewing process?
    - Review process of feedback - What information was effective/ineffective? Was the feedback specific? If not, how was it not specific?
    - What parts of the activities were geared to novice level skills, and how did each individual progress during the activity to more advanced skills?
    - What specifically were considered by the individuals involved to be advanced skills?

Additional Resources

McCallister, L. (1992). *I wish I'd said that! How to talk your way out of trouble and into success.* New York, NY: John Wiley and Sons.

Mortimer, J. A. (1983). *How to speak, how to listen.* New York, NY: Macmillan Publishing Company.

Rogers, C. R., & Roethlisberger, F. J. (1991). Barriers and gateways to communication. *Harvard Business Review,* Nov-Dec, pp.105-111.

Stewart, M., & Roter, D. (1989). *Communicating with medical patients.* London, England: Sage Publications.

Tannen, D. (1986). *That's not what I meant! How conversational style makes or breaks your relations with others.* New York, NY: William Morrow and Company.

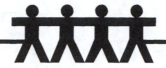

Chapter
Thirteen

Written Communication

Mary E. Muscari, PhD, CRNP, CS

Your remuneration has been currently augmented with a substantial aggregate of supplementary legal tender indelibly imprinted in single digit monetary units grossing one-hundred to the third power.

Do you understand that first sentence? Do you care?

Most likely you stopped reading due to confusion and frustration. That would be understandable but problematic because it means you just won $1,000,000.

Bad writing can really ruin your day.

Definition

Communication is the exchange of ideas. From cave walls to the Internet, humans have relied on written communication as a way of sharing information, a means of connection between two or more people. People communicate with each other almost every day. It would seem that we would have a clear understanding of each other's thoughts, ideas, and feelings, yet this frequently is not the case. Receivers often do not understand the sender's message. The communication process is more complicated than it appears (Sieh & Bretin, 1997), and good writers are made, not born.

Writing is a process. Notes, reports, and articles do not appear through wishful thinking. Even the best writers struggle through a complex process to achieve their end result. Their objective is to communicate an idea, either fact or fiction, in understandable terms. Unlike verbal communication, the written form allows for more preparation time, more permanence, and thus, more responsibility. Writers take full accountability for their words. Therefore, it is important that each word is carefully thought out before it is transcribed. You must think before you write.

Written communication is critical in interdisciplinary health care practice. You exchange ideas in a way that is clearly understood by all members of the health care team. The written form is quite variable and is used in charting, memos, letters, reports, and in more formal arenas such as research and publication. Each form is different in structure and style, but each is comparable in the basic necessities — clarity, accuracy, and brevity.

Significance

Did you understand that first sentence? Neither would your clients, your peers, or your colleagues. That first sentence may have been accurate and brief, but it certainly was not clear. You write to communicate, therefore your writing affects your professional relationships. Clients need to understand your written instructions. Peers need to understand your notes, and colleagues, your reports, papers, and research. Your writing is a permanent example of how you think — your knowledge level, your ability to analyze, and your ability to organize. Spoken words are carried in the wind, but written words are captured in plain view.

Client trust and compliance increase when given clear and concise written instructions. They are more confident in health care workers who give explicit directions. Peers respect the judgment of a fellow worker whose clinical notes are accurate, organized, and demonstrative of good judgment. Colleagues consult the provider who writes clear, yet thought provoking papers and research.

Background

Britton (1975) classified writing by its functions: expressive, transactional, and poetic. Expressive writing most resembles speaking with family and friends. It is closest to the writer's immediate thoughts and may be an end in itself, as in diary or letter writing. Expressive writing may also be shaped into more deliberate forms of communication, such as client assessments and progress notes. Transactional writing is used to communicate useful information to a reader. This form is used to communicate to a teacher through an essay or term paper, to colleagues in articles and research reports, and to prospective employers in resumés. Poetic writing is used in works of art like fiction and poetry. Despite the artistic dimensions of health care, this chapter will focus strictly on expressive and transactional forms of writing, with emphasis on the latter.

Gefvert (1988) notes that writing is a process that involves specific steps. However, it differs from other processes like house building. When contractors set out to build a house they usually begin with carefully drawn architectural plans. Writers usually discover what they are making during the process, and the various steps are done in different order by different writers. Some think, plan, and outline, others immediately start writing to get their ideas flowing. Although variations exist, certain activities occur in the process of good writing. They may not occur in order, and they may reoccur and overlap, but each is an important part of the process:

- *A Starting Point:* Everything must have a beginning. There is a question to answer, a problem to solve, or an idea to explore. Sometimes you pick the topic; most times it is assigned, although you usually have to angle it or use your own point of view.
- *Discovery:* The discovery of ideas or facts is part of every writing process.

- *Incubation and Illumination:* Most writers need to leave time for gestation or incubation, time when the conscious mind rests and the unconscious mind works. Illumination is the product of this activity.
- *Selecting:* Once you have thought about your subject and researched as many ideas as possible, you must choose your central idea and its supporting details.
- *Planning and Arranging:* This is where you decide the writing method and order that is best for your purpose. It may include outlining, it may not. You need to decide what works for you.
- *Writing a First Draft:* The first draft may come before or after selecting and arranging. It may come before or after the researching of ideas. However, at some point you need to put your notes into a logical order. This is not the time to worry about grammar and spelling.
- *Revising:* Now you can worry about grammar and spelling. Revision includes rewriting and editing. You rewrite to enhance the effectiveness of your sentences, noting arrangement, clarity, and style. You edit to correct grammar, spelling, punctuation, and usage.

Developing Written Communication Skills

General Guidelines

1. *Write, Write, Write.* Writing is a skill and a craft; therefore, like clinical skills, it requires both knowledge and practice. The good news is that most of you have been practicing writing skills long before entering college. The bad news is that you may have picked up some bad habits along the way. The great news is that you can still learn to write well and enjoy doing it.

2. *Read.* Read well-written charts, sample term papers, and articles. Study them for accuracy, clarity, and brevity. Ask yourself: "How did this writer clearly explain so much factual information in such few words? Then re-read the written piece to find your answer — the writer knew the subject matter, stayed focused, and used more nouns and verbs than adjectives and adverbs. Reading itself helps writing. Every well-written article, chapter, or book is a lesson in structure, style, grammar, and punctuation. You could also read about writing. Several excellent books exist on various aspects of writing. Check the reference section of your library or bookstore. Magazines such as *Writer's*

Digest and *The Writer* offer suggestions that are helpful for all levels of writers and writing. These can be found in most major bookstore magazine sections. Subscription information is given at the end of this chapter.

3. *Ask for Help.* Ask your teacher or go to your institution's learning center. Seek assistance from a respected preceptor, mentor, or clinician. Many of them have excellent writing skills, especially in expressive forms, and most are eager to help. Ask an author. Most faculty members write for publication; ask your advisor or another professor to mentor you or to at least point you in the right direction. You could even write to an author of one of your favorite professional articles or books and ask him or her about hi or her writing techniques.

Expressive Writing: Client Charting

The client chart or record is a permanent means of communication between health care providers. It facilitates coordinated planning and continuity of client care. The client chart also serves other purposes: it is the legal record for the health care agency and the professional staff responsible for the person's care; it provides the basis for evaluating the quality of care; it is a baseline for reviewing the effective use of client care services; and it furnishes data useful for research, education, and planning. Each agency selects from a variety of documentation systems by choosing one that best fits its needs. Systems include Problem-Oriented Charting, Focus Charting, Patient Outcome Charting, Problem Intervention Evaluation (PIE) Charting, and Charting by Exception (CBE). Some agencies use flow charts and computerized systems to save time, enhance monitoring of quality improvement issues, and make it easier to access client information (Smeltzer & Bare, 1996). Table 13-1 provides an example of a SOAP (Subjective, Objective, Assessment, Plan) note.

Regardless of the system used, good charting should be legally sound. It should reflect the process of the health care provided, a description of the client's status including assessments and diagnoses, expected client outcomes, and all provider interventions. Sieh and Bretin (1997) provide basic guidelines regarding the legalities and structure of charting:

- Use permanent ink and write in a legible manner.
- Never alter a chart after writing it. If you make a mistake, draw a single line through it and initial it.

Never erase in a chart.

- Do not chart for others. Chart only what you observe and do.
- Do not leave any space between your last entry and your signature; draw a line through unwritten space.
- Use only institutionally accepted abbreviations. Example: (L) unilateral sensory loss in UE & LE. Pt. is (R) dominant. Can wheel hemi w/c c min. difficulty; wears MOFO in shoe. Becky Young, Occupational Therapy Student, Class of 1999, University of Scranton, used with permission.
- Use correct spelling.
- Be objective, not subjective. Example: Exhibits impulsive behaviors indicating faulty judgment. Susan Relyea, Occupational Therapy Student, Class of 1999, University of Scranton, used with permission.
- Do not use chart to comment on other staff members.
- If you document a problem, document your intervention.
- Be accurate and clear, and use N/A for nonapplicable instead of leaving blank spaces.

The following is an excerpt from a client assessment written by a junior nursing student:

Chief Complaint: Low grade fever, mild dehydration & irritability

Present Illness: Three days prior to admission the patient became uncomfortable/irritable with feedings. Patient vomited the morning of 2-11-97 and had a fever. The child's appetite was noted as being decreased. There were no indications of nasal congestion, cough, rash, or sick contacts, according to the mother. Upon admission, the patient was sleepy with dry mucous membranes. He was easily awakened and resistant to examination. The rectal temp. was 100.4 F; W.T.: 13 lbs., 6 oz.; and respirations were 40/min. at rest. (Andrea Malone, Student Nurse, Class of 1998, University of Scranton, used with permission.)

The student documented the assessment in a clear and concise manner. Readers would not have difficulty understanding what was written.

Table 13-1

SAMPLE SOAP NOTE FROM STUDENT, WRITTEN

ACTIVITY ANALYSIS OF 40 Y/O FEMALE WITH (R) CVA

S: Prior Level of Function: (I) in ADLs & IADLs. *Home Set-up:* Lives with 2 children, 7y/o & 9y/o in 1 floor, 2 bed-room apt. Laundry room is located on 1st floor with 2 in. level Δ @ door threshold. Grocery store 4 blocks from home. *Work Situation:* Full-time librarian. Takes bus to/from work. No car. *Emotions & Attitudes:* Pt. became upset with frequent accidents because unable to get to toilet on time. Pt. Described as fiercely (I) & involved in neighborhood activities. *Leisure:* Pt. enjoys cooking, reading, going to son's sports events & spending time with family. *FH:* Hypercholesteremia.

O: Pt. had flaccid (L) trunk, UE & LE. (L) unilateral sensory loss, UE & LE, (L) ptosis. Pt. is right handed. *Perceptual & Cognitive Deficits:* exhibited impulsive behaviors to faulty judgement; difficulty with problem solving, learning new skills, concepts & generalization. Denial of (L) side, (L) visual deficit (hemianopsia), & motor apraxia. *Mobility:* Cannot maneuver w/c due to perceptual & cognitive & visual deficits. *ADLs:* Pt. Requires mod/max assistance.

A: Pt. Will require 4 wks inpatient rehab:
Problem list:

1. Dependent ADLs
2. Dependent ADL mobility
3. Flaccid (L) trunk
4. (L) unilateral sensory loss UE & LE
5. Perceptual & cognitive deficits
6. (L) visual field deficit
7. Motor apraxia

   Long-term goals:

   1. Return to prior level of function.
   2. Return home within 4 wks.
   3. (I) ADLs within 8 wks.
   4. Increase perceptual and cognitive capabilities within 4 wks.
   5. Return to work within 6 wks.
   6. Ambulate with walker within 3 months
   7. Resume child care responsibilities within 8 wks.

   Short-term goals:

   1. All transfers with minimal assist.
   2. Min. Assist with ADLs.
   3. Increase problem-solving, learning, concept formation & generalization.
   4. Increase (L) trunk control.
   5. Increase (L) unilateral sensation in UE & LE with tactile activities.
   6. Develop compensatory techniques for (L) hemianopsia

P: *BID:* Transfer training, LLE & LUE AROM exercises, visual tracking for hemianopsia. *OD:* Cognitive retraining, walker practice. *PRN:* Address safety awareness.

Written by Lauren Cavanaugh, Occupational Therapy Student, Class of 1999, University of Scranton, Scranton, PA (Used with permission).

Transactional Writing: Formal Papers and Manuscripts

Writing is a process that has a beginning, a middle, and an end. That process begins with the formulation of an idea and ends with the polished paper or manuscript.

Ideas. Thousands of papers are written every month, and each started with an idea. Ideas are thoughts, notions, and plans that come from many sources including clinical sites, formal and informal discussions, readings, and even personal experience. Ideas arise from frustration, desperation, and even elation, as every idea is sparked by some emotion. Passionate writers are more driven to complete the process.

The idea is the base of the article. Therefore it must be strong enough to support a complete manuscript. It must be clear, interesting, and useful. An idea is useful if the reader can extract something practical in the way of knowledge or skills. It must be meaningful. Homelessness, functional activities, and children with cancer are all ideas, useful starting points for an article.

Focusing the Idea. Many students conceptualize ideas that are too general, causing them to incorporate excess information in their papers. This usually results from overeagerness, fear of "missing something important," lack of organization, or the simple unawareness that focusing is important. For example, a student may attempt to write a 10 page paper addressing every historical, sociological, physical, and psychological factor related to homelessness. Excess information topples the idea, resulting in a domino effect of confusion and frustration for the reader. That leads to a low grade from the professor or a rejection letter from an editor.

An idea should be focused, i.e., it should be a specific topic. Suggested ways to improve focusing include brief literature reviews; discussions with classmates, peers, family, and friends; audio-taping ideas as they come to mind; journal writing; and random acts of writing. These all serve to promote focusing.

- The brief literature review provides focal points for ideas. See how other writers focused on specific topics. This is critical if you are trying to get published because it provides an overview of what has recently been written on a topic. Editors are unlikely to print recently published topics, unless the writer provides a unique approach. For example, if one journal recently covered meal preparation for clients with chronic schizophrenia, focus yours on meal preparation for clients who are recovering from strokes. Thinking about different approaches to the same general idea is another way of getting focused, and it could get you published.

- Never devalue the usefulness of a conversation. Professional writers get many an idea this way, and so can you. Well-read and clinically strong peers can pinpoint important topics, especially during impromptu discussions. Friends and family inundate you with health-related questions—turn one of them into a paper.

- Audio-taping works best for people who need to capture their fleeting thoughts. A pocket-sized, voice-activated cassette recorder fits easily in a pocket or purse and is readily available when ideas rush to mind.

- Journal or diary writing provides written accounts of daily observations and conversations from client contacts, peer discussions, and lectures. Somewhere in there is a well-focused topic just waiting to be written.

- Free-form writing is similar to audio-taping because you record your immediate thoughts. Today's gibberish could be tomorrow's award winning article.

Whatever the method, the result must be a focused idea, e.g., creative meal preparation for the elderly, oral care for preschoolers with leukemia, health problems of the rural homeless.

Developing the Idea. Ideas must be developed and expanded without losing focus. Idea development may include demographics, historical perspectives, etiologies, specific disorders, symptoms, multidiscipline involvement, psychosocial factors, and interventions. Ethical, political, and legal elements provide interesting viewpoints for controversial ideas, such as providing confidential health care to adolescent clients, or the amount of required supervision for licensed and unlicensed personnel.

Use brief outlines and note-taking to expand ideas. This outline usually bears little resemblance to the final paper, however it helps the development process. Outlining also aids the researching process, which could be very tedious for popular topics.

Researching the Idea. The idea grows through research. The library is a good place to start. Unless otherwise specified, literature reviews concentrate on primary material (works by original authors) from the last 3 to 5 years and the "classics." Classics are generally books that stand the test of time due to their authorship, content, or both. The indices, both bound (Nursing and Allied Health [CINHAL]) and CD-ROM (CINHAL), are valuable. Use the reference lists at the end of articles. When all else fails, the key library resource is the reference librarian, revered by writers as the ultimate resource.

Experts are invaluable data sources and can be found as near as your professor or colleague. Experts are passionate about their areas of expertise and eager to provide information and resources. The World Wide Web holds an abundance of health related information and allows access to hospital and university home pages, libraries, and discussion networks. Be careful not to drown while surfing, the information can get overwhelming at times.

Literature review findings vary. Some topics have endless material, others nearly none. Allocate sufficient time for research to ensure that you have extracted or exhausted the material you need. You can record your findings on index cards, notebooks, computer, or audio-tapes. Whatever the method used, carefully note the source to give proper reference credit and to enable retrieval if needed later.

Audience. Once you know what to write, you need to know who you are writing for, i.e., the reader or audience. Most professional articles are slanted toward specific audiences — occupational therapists, pediatric nurses — all of whom are at specific levels. These include experience levels (students, new graduates, and experienced practitioners), focus areas (practice, education), practice levels (generalist or specialty/advanced practice), and/or practice areas (psychosocial, pediatrics, home health). It is easier to begin a paper with an audience in mind. If the audience is not specified, a common trait in term paper assignments, ask the professor for an audience or write it to an audience of your own level.

If you are writing a manuscript for publication, audience selection rests with you. It may be a conscious choice (writing a physical assessment article for advanced primary care nurses versus hospital based generalists) or a natural result of the topic (meal preparation for clients with chronic schizophrenia in group home settings). Whatever the selection, keep the audience in mind by continuously thinking, "What do they need or want to know about this topic?" This will assist you with content selection, organization, and writing style.

Selecting a Title. Once you are comfortable with your topic, start writing. A good place to start is the title. Give your paper a working title, something to keep you focused, such as "Creative meal preparation for the elderly," or "Oral care for preschoolers with leukemia." The title can be changed once the paper is completed.

Structure. Papers and manuscripts are written in a logical sequence from start to finish. You can institute structure by using outlines or note cards. Detailed outlines create and maintain structure and pave the way to a completed first draft. The detailed outline is more focused and

content-laden than the preliminary outline. Each section of the detailed outline contains commentary from the literature or experience.

Computerized and index note cards have their own advantages. Computerized notes can be easily transferred into the first draft, especially for persons who can develop papers right on the computer. Index cards can be easily arranged for a full visual effect and they can be rearranged on a table, mat, or posterboard until they form a logical sequence. They are also the logical choice for those of us new to both writing and computers.

The First Draft. New or not, all potential writers must overcome the urge to escape the computer. Even professional writers fear blank screens, failure, and rejection. Sooner or later, you will have to sit down and write. Get your words down on paper or on the monitor—you can correct them later. Long-time screenwriter Art Arthur declared that there were two secrets to becoming a successful screenwriter; his words are useful to all writers: "Don't get it right, get it written" and "The seat of the pants to the seat of the chair" (Hauge, 1991).

Writing takes time and energy, therefore you need to find the best times with the least interruptions (early morning, late night, when your significant other is out, when your kids are in school, after you walk the dog). Blank screens happen — keep writing. Keep your ideas flowing, no matter how badly they read. This is a first draft; write first, edit later.

The lead paragraph is critical. If it is dull, unclear, or poorly written, why should the reader keep reading? The lead should be interesting, and it should convey the purpose and tone for the rest of the article. It should clearly state what the article is all about:

The word "homeless" conjures up pictures of city streets laced with disheveled beggars and bag ladies. No one pictures the rural homeless or their plight. Yet, homelessness is a fact in rural America, and the rural homeless face numerous health-related problems.

The lead paragraph is usually the most difficult to write, but it gives focus. You can rewrite it when the manuscript is polished.

Write the body of the first draft according to the outline. Do not write a jumbled list of annotated references. Use your "voice" as a critical element of style to project a proficient analysis of your content. Shout, "I know what I'm talking about." The article's tone should be one of competence and authority, with you analyzing and/or critiquing the literature as you present it. No one "hears" a voiceless article.

More is synonymous with better. Most papers are about 8 to 16 pages in length. However, you may include information in your first draft and remove it when you polish. It is always better to keep writing than to stare at a blank screen.

The conclusion style depends upon the content. Conclusions may be circular, linear or summative. In circular conclusions, the writer refers back to the beginning of the article. In linear endings, the writer makes suggestions, like practitioner implications or research ideas. Many writers simply end with a summation of the manuscript's contents. Regardless of style, conclusions should be interesting and stimulating. Do not leave the reader feeling abandoned after enjoying a paper or manuscript about an interesting subject.

Rewriting. Few get it right the first time. Writers rely on revisions to enhance and reorganize their work. Revisions are best done several days after completing the first draft to get a fresh perspective — therefore, do not write term papers the night before they are due! You may rewrite directly on the computer or on hard copy (printout). Either way, revisions are essential to ensure a finished, polished paper or manuscript.

Murray (1995) describes seven critical processes for revision: focus, collect, shape, order, develop, voice, and edit:

1. Focus: There should be one, single dominant purpose to the paper. The focus should be clear enough to explain the article in one sentence. For example, this article explains techniques to create methods of meal planning for the elderly.
2. Collect: The paper represents a collection of accurate, specific and significant data. Make sure that your paper is filled with the concise analysis of pertinent research data and significant clinical information.
3. Shape: The paper should be written in a form that is familiar to the reader. Most papers are written in the narrative form using a logical sequence.
4. Order: Disorganized outlines lead to chaotic drafts and require restructuring during revision. Your paper should be written in a coherent, sequential manner. When reading it, you should be able to excerpt your outline. Proper sequencing can be simple. Using the example of the oral care for children with leukemia, the writer could give logical order by progressing from assessment to intervention.
5. Develop: Your writing should reflect you as a writer who provides information that is specific, accurate, and interesting. Do not regurgitate literature; revitalize it.
6. Voice: Readers should be able to detect the person behind the article. You want to stimulate and challenge your readers. Carry them forward by the energy of the flow of the article.
7. Edit: The paper should be clear, accurate, and specific. It should flow properly and have meaning. Format it properly (many health care programs and journals use APA Style, the style suggested by the *Publication Manual of the American Psychological Association*). Avoid clichés and jargon, use the active voice, cut out unnecessary words, assure proper spelling and grammar, and check the accuracy of references.

Nothing is sacred; eliminate or edit anything that does not contribute something substantial (Pratt, 1997). You may need to write multiple drafts before reaching the final product. However, the revision process can be a rewarding experience as you nurture the manuscript to maturity.

Getting Your Manuscript Published. The emphasis here is the word *manuscript*. Term papers are rarely in publishable format and will most likely be returned by a very unhappy editor. If you want to publish your term paper, rewrite for publication. However, polished manuscripts deserve homes other than circular files. They deserve the good home of a professional journal.

Journal selection depends on the targeted audience. Narrow the choice to journals that cater to your targeted audience characteristics (experience level, focus area, practice area, and practice level) and then read several issues to study writing style and format. Regard the audience characteristics to decide which journal is appropriate. For example, if the oral care article is aimed at staff nurses, it is unsuitable for an occupational therapy journal. Likewise, if your hand skills for preschoolers article is aimed at occupational therapists, it is unsuitable for a nursing journal.

Once possible journals are selected, review what each has published in the past 2 years to avoid duplication and to get a feel of the journal's writing style. Then select the journal that is most similar to your own style.

Most journals provide "Author Guidelines" or "Information for Authors." These are comprehensive explanations of the journal's expectations for manuscript content, format, and submission. Many journals list their guidelines in each or specific issue(s), others will send them at your request.

Follow the guidelines carefully. They provide information on reference style, page length, spacing, margins, titles, abstracts, organization, and displays (tables, graphs,

Table 13-2

SAMPLE QUERY LETTER

Institution
Department
Street Address
City, State, Zip Code
Telephone Number with Area Code

Editor's Name
Editor's Specific Title
Journal Title
Street Address
City, State, Zip Code

Dear Mr./Mrs. ....:

I write to inquire if you would be interested in reviewing my manuscript, "Title," for possible publication in your journal, "Journal Title". The manuscript details are... (two to four sentences describing contents of article).

As a ... (brief description of your credentials to write article).

The manuscript is ready for submission. A disk copy is also available in either WordPerfect 6.1 (or whatever word processing software was used) or ASCII, and will be sent at your request.

Thank you for your time and consideration. I look forward to hearing from you.

Sincerely,

Name
Title

figures, etc.). Manuscripts that disregard guidelines will either be rejected or sent back for considerable revision.

Many journals accept unsolicited (not requested by editor) manuscripts, however, you can query first. The query letter is written to see if the editor is interested in reviewing the manuscript for possible publication (Table 13-2). Write a short, one-page letter that briefly describes your manuscript, concisely characterizes your credentials to write the manuscript, and gives the status of your article's progress. Address the editor by name and proper title, both of which are found on the masthead (list of editor and staff names) in the first few pages of the latest issue, or through telephone correspondence with journal personnel.

Query letters save you time, energy, and postage. The editor may be disinterested in your manuscript due to impending publication of a similar topic or its lack of fit with the journals' needs. In that case, the unsolicited man-

uscript will probably not be read and may sit on an editor's desk for some time. Your query letter is more likely to receive a faster reply. If the topic is undesirable, then you can query another journal. You may query more than one journal at a time, but you may not submit the same manuscript to more than one journal at the same time. Use caution with multiple query submissions — if more than one journal is interested, and your first choice ultimately rejects you, you must then go back to a journal that you turned down. Most journals respond to queries in 2 to 6 weeks. If you do not receive a response after 6 weeks, call the editor and question the query's status.

Once you receive a positive response, send the final draft, along with a title page, the required number of readable, smudge-proof copies, and a cover letter. Your cover letter should thank the editor for considering your article for review, and it should solicit suggestions, comments, and criticisms. Send your "prized possession" by

Table 13-3

SAMPLE FROM A STUDENT TERM PAPER

Written for General Public (Audience)

Introductory Paragraph:

Planning a night out with some friends or a romantic dinner with your love? Chances are, no matter how you spend your evening, alcohol will be available and most likely consumed. Alcohol has found a permanent place in our society, and the ill effects of alcohol on a developing fetus have been known throughout history, dating back as far as Aristotle and even the Old Testament. Although warnings to avoid alcohol during pregnancy have been documented for years, many pregnant women are still unclear of the effects of alcohol on the growing fetus. Millions of women carelessly consume alcohol during pregnancy, and as a result their children suffer. There is a common myth that a minimal amount of alcohol during pregnancy is fine. Others believe that a little every now and then is good for the mother and baby. But study after study has shown the damage of alcohol during pregnancy. Alcohol has been found to cause an endless list of birth complications, and pregnant women need to know!

Written by Daria Mills, Nursing Student, Class of 1998, University of Scranton, Scranton, PA (Used with permission).

either certified or registered mail, with a return receipt, so that you know it arrived safely. Do not call to ask if the editor received it.

When the manuscript reaches the journal, it is analyzed by a panel of reviewers who judge your manuscript on the basis of its usefulness, timeliness, and writing style. Reviewers then give the editor their comments and suggestions, including publication acceptance and revision suggestions. The review process can take up to 6 months or more; call if it takes longer. When the editor responds with a letter of interest, it almost always asks for revisions. Editors and reviewers make suggestions to create better articles, not to aggravate you.

Return your revised copy to the editor for final approval. Once approved, you await the galley proofs (the printed copy in its typeset form). Galley proofs arrive just prior to publication; you review these for correctness and make minimal revisions.

Now you can either sit back and wait to see your name in print or you can start on your next article. Success breeds more success. Table 13-3 is an excerpt from a student paper targeted toward a general audience, as per her assignment.

Levels of Development

Due to the nature of written communication, students and clinicians may be at varying levels of development at the same time. They may be at the intermediate level for expressive writing and at the novice level for transactional writing. Some may have an artistic streak and perform as experts in poetic writing. Regardless of level, there is always room for improvement.

Novice

Beginning novices have no experience in the tasks that they need to perform and are given situations in terms of objective attributes such as measurements and deadlines. Rules must be followed and behaviors are extremely limited and inflexible. Advanced beginners have coped with real situations enough to learn their aspects, the global characteristics that can be learned only through experience. The ability to communicate complex subject matter depends on previous experience with that subject matter (Benner, 1984).

Novices frequently stumble over legions of grammar and punctuation rules, dangling participles, and confusing commas and semi-colons. They occasionally write clear sentences, but more frequently cloud their topics with excessive jargon and pompous phrases in hopes of impressing their professor.

Jargon becomes a double-edged sword as novices struggle to learn new terminology and how, when, and where to use it. Charting is occasionally erroneous and sometimes humorous (describing a bedsore on the *cervix* of a *male* client). Term papers are typically filled with regurgitated literature and extraneous information as novices frequently lose focus on their topic and boldly go where no instructor wants them to go. Medical dictionaries and thesauruses are student writers' best friends and worst enemies.

Once novices progress through experience, they are able to better communicate ideas and opinions clearly and concisely in writing papers, notes, and reports. They also begin to tackle complex subject matter and present it in a clear manner, using correct punctuation and grammar more frequently.

Apprentice

Professionals who face the same situations for 2 to 3 years typically demonstrate competence. Competence develops when clinicians see their actions in terms of long-term goals. Plans are based on considerable conscious, abstract, and analytical contemplation of the problem. Competent clinicians lack the speed and flexibility of the proficient professional, however, they have a feeling of mastery. Eventually there is efficiency and organization, after what seems to be great effort. The proficient clinician is the one who most frequently notes deterioration or client problems prior to explicit changes. However, this is the person who regresses to the competent level when faced with novelty or the demand for an analytic, procedural description.

Apprentices should be able to write concise clinical notes that can be clearly understood by any health-related discipline. Knowledge and experience should be at a level where the writer is able to chart with little preparation, unless faced with a complex situation. Transactional writings should be clear, with ideas and opinions communicated effectively 75 to 95% of the time. The apprentice is able to write a professional article with assistance from a seasoned writer or editor.

Expert

Expert performers no longer rely on analytic principles to connect situations to actions. Due to enormous experiential backgrounds, experts have an intuitive grasp of situations and the ability to zone in on problems without wasting time. However, expertise is not always descriptive because the expert operates from a deep understanding of total situations. Comments may be as nondescriptive as, "It doesn't feel right" or "I just know it." Experts may also respond to hypothetical questions with responses such as, "It all depends."

Expert clinicians can also provide consultative services for other clinicians, both inside and outside their disciplines. They are very effective in detecting early changes and making recommendations. In the past, many experts had little opportunity to compare and develop consensus on their observations. Now with the advent of the Internet, experts are free to network around the world.

Written forms of communication are clear and concise. Clinical charting excels in this, despite depth of understanding and abstraction level. Experts consistently put clinical observations into a clearly understood written format. Writers at the expert level also engage in formal written communication through article writing and research reports. Complex subject matter is communicated in a clear and concise manner with little outside direction. However, most experts seek the opinions of other seasoned writers so that they may enhance their work.

References

Bean, J. (1996). *Engaging ideas: The professor's guide to integrating writing, critical thinking, and active learning in the classroom.* San Francisco, CA: Jossey-Bass Publishers.

Benner, P. (1984). *From novice to expert.* Melona Park, CA: Addison-Wesley Publishing Co.

Britton, J. (1975). *The development of writing abilities.* London, England: Macmillian Education.

Hauge, M. (1991). *Writing screenplays that sell.* New York, NY: Harper Collins Publishers.

Murray, D. (1995). *The craft of revision,* 2nd Edition. Fort Worth, TX: Harcourt Brace Publishers.

Muscari, M. (1998). Do the write thing: Writing the clinically focused article. *Journal of Pediatric Health Care, 12,* 236-41.

Sieh, A., & Bretin, L. (1997). *The nurse communicates.* Philadelphia, PA: WB Saunders Co.

Smeltzer, S., & Bare, B. (1996). *Brunner and Suddarth's textbook of medical-surgical nursing,* 8th Edition. Philadelphia, PA: Lippincott, 29-30.

Exercises for Written Communication

Chose a clinically-related topic other than the ones noted in this chapter. The topic should be discipline-specific, as well as one that sparks your interest. Explain the topic by writing the following (you must use the same topic for each assignment):

1. A one-page letter to a friend or family member.

2. A two-page memo to a peer.

3. A list of instructions for a client.

4. A formal paper (term paper or manuscript). For this one, follow the guidelines suggested in this chapter, from focusing your idea, through outlining a first draft, to a polished paper.

5. Compare assignments 1 through 4. How and why are they similar? How and why are they different? What language and voice did you use? Was one assignment more clear than the others?

Additional Resources

Books

American Psychological Association. (1994). *Publication Manual of the American Psychological Association,* 4th Edition. Washington, DC: American Psychological Association.

Gerard, P. (1996). *Creative nonfiction: Researching and crafting the stories of real life.* Cincinnati, OH: Story Press.

Keyes, R. (1995). *The courage to write.* New York, NY: Henry Holt and Company.

Maloy, T. (1996). *The internet research guide.* New York, NY: Allworth Press.

Murray, D. (1995). *The craft of revision,* Second Edition. Fort Worth, TX: Harcourt Brace Publishers.

Strunk, W., & White, E. (1979). *The elements of style,* 3rd Edition. New York, NY: MacMillan.

Walvoord, B. (1986). *Helping students write well: A guide for teachers in all disciplines.* New York, NY: The Modern Language Association of America.

Williams, J. (1990). *Style: Toward clarity and grace.* Chicago, IL: The University of Chicago Press.

Magazines

Writer's Journal
Val-Tech Publishing, Inc.
P. O. Box 25376
St. Paul, MN 55125

The Writer, Inc.
120 Boylston Street
Boston, MA 02116-4615
888-273-8214

Writer's Digest
Box 2123
Harlan, IA 51593
800-333-0133

Organizations

For those interested in writing for publication or just support, check your school or local paper for writer's groups. If there are none listed, start one. Collect a few well-intentioned friends, talk to a faculty member, or call a writer for assistance.

Other

1. Ask a faculty member to mentor you.
2. Use the college learning resource center.
3. Ask the reference librarian for sources.
4. Use the university writing center.

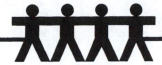

Part Three

Measuring Up: The Professional Development Assessment

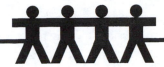

Chapter Fourteen

Development of the Instrument, and its Academic and Clinical Applications

Jack Kasar,
PhD, OTR/L

Assessing and growing professional behaviors in health care students and practitioners is an important and timely undertaking. There have been a number of presentations at conferences and meetings underscoring the significance of professionalism, and a limited but steady number of articles in the literature. This section will focus on the development of a tool to assess professional behaviors, and academic and clinical applications using the instrument, together with some suggestions on how to enhance the behaviors. The information should prove useful to health care professions students, particularly when students become practitioners and eventually educators.

Assessment of Professional Values and Behaviors

There are a limited number of assessments that have looked at professional values and behaviors, with the larger majority having come from the nursing profession. Eddy, Elfrink, Weis, & Schank (1994) compared ratings of faculty with that of students, of the importance of professional nursing values embodied in the Professional Nursing Behavior Instrument. They found that faculty rated the importance of behaviors significantly higher than did students, and that faculty valued equality, human dignity, and freedom greater than students. Some of the other behavioral categories assessed were altruism, justice, and truth. An earlier study,using a survey instrument also compared faculty and student ratings of values and again found that faculty ratings of professional values were higher than student ratings (Thurston, Flood, Shupe, & Gerald, 1989). Ratings of personal values were similar between faculty and students, which supports the notion that individuals are attracted to a profession by the beliefs they perceive it to represent, and how well-suited they believe their skills and abilities are to that field.

A self-rating behavioral inventory to assess professional behaviors in nurses was developed by Miller, Adams and Beck (1993). Their inventory took a broad view of professionalism and considered aspects such as educational background, community service, communication and publication, and research involvement. They also looked at adherence to the code of ethics, involvement in professional organizations, self-regulation, and use and development of theory. The Professionalism Inventory that they developed was used in a study of hospital nurse executives and middle managers in 10 western states (Adams, Miller, & Beck, 1996). It was determined that nurse executives rated themselves higher than middle managers for all categories of professional behavior except for knowledge of the code of ethics and autonomy.

The Professional Self Description Form was used in a study in Sweden to examine the perception of professional self among OTs (Gullberg, Olsson, Alenfelt, Ivarsson, & Nilsson, 1994). The form is a self-administered, paper-and-pencil, seven-point Likert scale, comprised of 19 items related to concepts thought to be inherent in professional functioning. Some of the items included in the scale are drive, reliability, flexibility, persistence, resourcefulness, and sensitivity. Factor analysis of the 19 items yielded five factors: problem-solving ability, empathy, working capacity, professionalism, and management. These factors were deemed essential to functioning in the role of the professional occupational therapist in Sweden.

Opacich and Hughes (1990) examined professional behaviors in OT graduates during the first year of employment. A scale was used which looked at 17 attributes, and rated students from poor to superior. Some of the behaviors assessed included judgment, leadership, technical repertoire, and professional identity. A Likert-type scale was developed by Kautzmann (1984) to provide feedback on professional behavior during Level I fieldwork. The types of behaviors that were evaluated were more definitive and specific, for example, participating with the supervising therapist in clinical problem-solving, and appropriately asking for information or help.

Development of the Instrument

While a few assessments have been developed and applied to circumstances within certain professions, what was needed was a way to systematically, somewhat objectively, focus attention on the importance of professional behaviors, both in the classroom and in the clinic. The *Professional Development Assessment* (Table 14-1) was designed to address that need.

The assessment was primarily constructed to get a handle on a way to provide feedback to students on the development of their professional behaviors, and as a means for them to look at their level of functioning through self-evaluation. The first version contained 10 categories: dependability, professional presentation, initiative, empathy, cooperation, organization, clinical reasoning, supervisory process, verbal communication, and written communication (Kasar, 1994). The behavioral categories were valued and deemed important for students and practitioners to have, as suggested by an informal survey of students, clinical supervisors, and academicians in the

Northeast and Mid-Atlantic states, over a 5-year period. The information was gathered during annual visits to clinics and regional meetings with educators. The categories were rated on a four-point scale, with four (4) being consistently shown, and one (1) being rarely evidenced. The total possible score ranged from a low of 10 to a high of 40. The 10 items are by no means all inclusive, and any one item has many facets and aspects to it, and is not simplistic or discreet. The goal was to construct an assessment that was relatively quick and easy to use by both academicians and clinicians, and that would provide useful information to students.

The assessment was initially used in the OT Practice courses in the junior and senior years of the 4-year OT program at Elizabethtown College, and included the areas of pediatrics, psychosocial rehabilitation, and physical rehabilitation. Students were rated by the academic instructor for the portion of the course related to lectures, labs, seminars, and field trips. The same tool was used by clinical supervisors for Level I fieldwork to rate students on how they functioned in the clinical setting (these were initial clinicals concurrent with academic coursework). The scores from both settings were averaged, with the resultant figure accounting for 20% of the final course grade. This was enough to get appropriate attention from students, but generally not enough to cause them to fail in the course. However, if their overall performance was marginal to begin with, it prevented them from getting the minimum grade of C that was required in all OT and related courses. On the other hand, students who clearly demonstrated the requisite professional behaviors were positively reinforced by having their course grade bolstered. Students were oriented to and given a copy of the assessment in their Level I Fieldwork Manual, and were strongly encouraged to read and review it. Clinical supervisors reviewed the manual and the assessment prior to the clinical experience in a group session at the school.

The initial form of the assessment, while somewhat quantifiable, needed the behavioral categories to be more specific and detailed, and the rating scale options to be better delineated. The original assessment was developed into its current form in the summer of 1994 and revised in 1996 (Kasar, Clark, Watson, & Pfister, 1996). The *Professional Development Assessment* retained the basic 10 categories, but three behavioral descriptors were developed for each of the items. The intent was to make the assessment more objective and quantifiable, and to arrange the descriptors in a hierarchical fashion from least to more difficult/complex behavior. An example of the

Table 14-1

PROFESSIONAL DEVELOPMENT ASSESSMENT©

Name: _____

Evaluator (other than self): _____

Date: _____

Instructions: For each professional behavior, review the descriptors and rate 1 through 4 by circling the selected number.

Rating Scale:
1. Rarely (50% or less of the time).
2. Occasionally (50 to 75% of the time).
3. Frequently (75 to 95% of the time).
4. Consistently (95% or more of the time).

1. Dependability as demonstrated by:

a. Being on time for classes, work, meetings.	1	2	3	4
b. Handing in assignments, papers, reports, and notes when due.	1	2	3	4
c. Following through with commitments and responsibilities.	1	2	3	4

Comments:

2. Professional Presentation as demonstrated by:

a. Presenting oneself in a manner that is accepted by peers, clients, and employers.	1	2	3	4
b. Using body posture and affect that communicates interest or engaged attention.	1	2	3	4
c. Displaying a positive attitude towards becoming a professional.	1	2	3	4

Comments:

3. Initiative as demonstrated by:

a. Showing an energetic, positive, and motivated manner.	1	2	3	4
b. Self-starting projects, tasks, and programs.	1	2	3	4
c. Taking initiative to direct own learning.	1	2	3	4

Comments:

4. Empathy as demonstrated by:

a. Being sensitive and responding to the feelings and behaviors of others.	1	2	3	4
b. Listening to and considering the ideas and opinions of others.	1	2	3	4
c. Rendering assistance to all individuals without bias or prejudice.	1	2	3	4

Comments:

5. Cooperation as demonstrated by:

a. Working effectively with other individuals.	1	2	3	4
b. Showing consideration for the needs of the group.	1	2	3	4
c. Developing group cohesiveness by assisting in the development of the knowledge and awareness of others.	1	2	3	4

Comments:

Table 14-1 continued

PROFESSIONAL DEVELOPMENT ASSESSMENT©

6. Organization as demonstrated by:

a.	Prioritizing self and tasks.	1	2	3	4
b.	Managing time and materials to meet program requirements.	1	2	3	4
c.	Using organization skills to contribute to the development of others.	1	2	3	4

Comments:

7. Clinical Reasoning as demonstrated by:

a.	Using an inquiring or questioning approach in class and clinic.	1	2	3	4
b.	Analyzing, synthesizing, and interpreting information.	1	2	3	4
c.	Giving alternative solutions to complex issues and situations.	1	2	3	4

Comments:

8. Supervisory Process as demonstrated by:

a.	Giving and receiving constructive feedback.	1	2	3	4
b.	Modifying performance in response to meaningful feedback.	1	2	3	4
c.	Operating within the scope of one's own skills and seeking guidance when needed.	1	2	3	4

Comments:

9. Verbal Communication as demonstrated by:

a.	Verbally interacting in class and clinic.	1	2	3	4
b.	Sharing perceptions and opinions with clarity and quality of content.	1	2	3	4
c.	Verbalizing opposing opinions with constructive results.	1	2	3	4

Comments:

10. Written Communication as demonstrated by:

a.	Writing clear sentences.	1	2	3	4
b.	Communicating ideas and opinions clearly and concisely in writing papers, notes, and reports.	1	2	3	4
c.	Communicating complex subject matter clearly and concisely in writing, with correct punctuation and grammar.	1	2	3	4

Comments:

third category, Initiative, with behavioral descriptors listed is as follows:

3. Initiative as demonstrated by:

a. Showing an energetic, positive, and motivated manner.

b. Self-starting projects, tasks and programs.

c. Taking initiative to direct own learning.

Several OT programs at the assistant and professional level field-tested the instrument and assisted in the collection of data for initial validity and reliability studies (see assessment in this chapter and in the Appendix). The assessment was also piloted with students in several other disciplines at Mount Aloysius College, including nursing, radiological technology, and medical technology. The student self-ratings were similar to the OT students.

Initial Validity and Reliability Information

The *Professional Development Assessment* was used initially with students in a 2-year occupational therapy assistant program at Mount Aloysius College (n = 20), and a 4-year undergraduate occupational therapy program at the University of Scranton (n = 35). The actual number of students in each group was considerably higher, but those with any missing data were excluded from the analysis. The students self-assessed using the form at the beginning of their first semester in school. A descriptive analysis of their summed scores for the 10 categories of professional behaviors showed a similar ranking between schools (Table 14-2). Dependability, empathy, cooperation, and professional presentation were ranked highest. Verbal communication and clinical reasoning were ranked lowest. Initiative, however, was ranked fifth for the Mount Aloysius students and ninth for the University of Scranton students. This might reflect the fact that the students from the 4-year program were traditional age, just out of high school and lower in motivation, as compared to older, non-traditional students found in the 2-year program. The older students are making many sacrifices to attend school, with families, part-time jobs, etc., and therefore are much more serious about their education. Also for all categories, the Mount Aloysius students rated themselves higher, which might again reflect the fact that they are older, more mature, aware, confident of their behaviors, and generally possess more life experience.

The behavioral descriptors for the most part seemed to be hierarchically arranged from least to most difficult/complex behavior. Also, it would be anticipated that more students scored themselves higher on the least difficult behavior and lower on the more complex behavior, on the four-point scale.

Concurrent with the initial use of the assessment by students in the two programs, 50 faculty in a variety of programs and 20 clinical supervisors at Mount Aloysius College, in addition to six members of the Curriculum Advisory Committee at the University of Scranton, were all asked to rate the behavioral descriptors as to whether they were valued, and important for students and practitioners to demonstrate. They also used a four-point scale to relatively rate the significance of the behaviors, with 4 being highly valued, and 1 having minimal value. The vast majority of professionals consistently rated most of the items as a 4, a few noted some as a 3, and hardly any 2 or 1 choices were selected. This lends support to the idea that the assessment taps behaviors that are deemed important for professionals to possess, and that are reflective of the behavioral categories.

A second class of new students at the two schools self-assessed using the form the next year, and a third school, the University of South Alabama (n = 21), which is a junior-level entry OT curriculum, was added to the study. The self-assessment of the University of Scranton students was almost identical to the first class of students, with the exception that initiative improved slightly and was now ranked eighth ahead of clinical reasoning. The students at Mount Aloysius College also rated themselves very similarly to the first class.

Pilot testing of the assessment was continued with students in the three programs, and a summary of the findings will now be presented. Using the form, a total of 76 students rated themselves at the start of their professional studies and again after a period of 1 to 2 years, depending on their respective programs. The characteristics of the entire sample at the time of the second self-assessment were as follows: mean age 24.3 years, with a range of ages from 19 to 52, and a median of 21; sex, male 18%, female 82%; years in school, 3, with a range of 2 to 4; ethnicity, Euro-American 98%, American Indian 1%, and Hispanic 1%. The three groups were characteristic of students at their particular institution, and were from predominantly middle-class backgrounds.

T-tests for paired samples were run for the sample of participants from each school and it was found that there was no significant difference between the 1st and 2nd self-assessment, reflective of consistency of the instrument over time. There was a significant difference among

Table 14-2

COMPARISON OF SUMMED SCORES AND RANK FOR THE BEHAVIORAL CATEGORIES

Professional Behavior	University of Scranton	Mount Aloysius College
1. Dependability	11.3 (1st)	11.6 (1st)
2. Professional Presentation	10.2 (4th)	10.8 (4th)
3. Initiative	9.0 (9th)	10.6 (5th)
4. Empathy	11.2 (2nd)	11.3 (2nd)
5. Cooperation	10.7 (3rd)	11.1 (3rd)
6. Organization	9.4 (7th)	10.3 (7th)
7. Clinical Reasoning	9.0 (8th)	9.5 (9th)
8. Supervisory Process	9.8 (5th)	10.3 (6th)
9. Verbal Communication	8.9 (10th)	9.3 (10th)
10. Written Communication	9.4 (6th)	9.8 (8th)

schools in tests of between-subjects effects, with F significant at the .050 level, but there was no interaction effect. A Pearson correlation was run on pretest and posttest scores and was found to be .48, which was statistically significantly different from zero (t = 4.75, p < .001, two-tailed test). When an r to Fisher's Zr and back to r conversion was performed, it gave a 95% confidence interval of .31 to .62, wherein the pretest scores accounted for 23% of the variance in the posttest scores (Kasar, 1997). This again lends support to the stability of the *Professional Development Assessment*.

The Coefficient Alpha for this group of students' scores was .65, which supports internal reliability. A correlation matrix was conducted on the ten professional behaviors, and out of a total of 45 correlations, 40 were significantly positively related. Only five of the correlations were not significant, overall suggesting that there is a correlation among the behaviors. A factor analysis was performed and two factors emerged, with a loading that was accounted for on factor 1 — 48.8% and factor 2 — 14.2%, for a total of 63.1% of the variance. The professional behaviors that were related to factor 1 were: initiative, organization, clinical reasoning, verbal communication, and written communication, which seems to comprise motivation, thinking, and communication skills. The professional behaviors related to factor 2 were: dependability, professional presentation, empathy, cooperation, and supervisory process, which seems to comprise responsibility, interacting, sensing, and feeling.

Finally, inter-rater reliability was conducted with the group of students from the University of South Alabama (n = 21) and three of the instructors who rated their behavior. The inter-rater reliability coefficient of the mean three raters was .74, again supporting reliability. As noted, this is an initial analysis on a small sample of students and faculty; however the results are promising and support the reliability and validity of the instrument. Additional studies with larger numbers of students, clinicians, and faculty need to be carried out.

Academic and Clinical Applications

The current version of the assessment has been used for the past several years with OT students in a developing, 4-year undergraduate program. On day one of the first occupational therapy introductory course during the first week of school, students self-assess using the *Professional Development Assessment*. During the first 2 years of the program, students are provided individual developmental feedback related to behavioral categories from the assessment, which is designed to facilitate enhancement of professional behaviors. Later, course instructors and clinical supervisors evaluate demonstration of the behaviors in the classroom and clinical settings, and then continue to compare their ratings with the students' self-assessment and encourage growth. Finally, employers rate graduates of the program, using the assessment, during the first year of employment.

Clinicians can also use the assessment tool to self-evaluate to encourage further development. Supervisors can use the measure to focus and assist staff in the areas in which they need to grow, and as part of an employee performance appraisal system.

Strategies for Developing Professional Behaviors

Program Planning

The mission of the Department of Occupational Therapy is in keeping with the University of Scranton Statement of Mission to prepare humanistically-trained professionals with a solid liberal arts and science foundation. The idea of developing professional behaviors did not occur in a vacuum, but rather grew as a natural extension of the mission of the school, department, and curriculum model. The goal of the program is to develop strong, generalist, entry-level therapists with the capacity for critical thinking, creative analysis, and clinical reasoning. Emphasis is placed on learning, the search for truth, and a sense of ethical responsibility in striving for personal growth and development. Attention is given to community service to enhance the personal and professional experience of students by providing the opportunity to use their skills and abilities to help others. The mission, curriculum model and goals could be found with some variations in most any health care professions program.

The curriculum is based on a frame of reference that is developmental, humanistic, and holistic in nature, and which emphasizes optimal function throughout the lifespan. Other courses are included in the general curriculum that facilitate professionalism, such as public speaking for verbal communication; ethics, philosophy, and theology for sensitivity and awareness of self and others (empathy); computer literacy course for telecommunications; and group dynamics for teamwork and cooperation.

The development of professional behaviors is specifically targeted by attempting to actualize and operationalize a number of the 12 educational goals for graduates of the program. In fact, the majority of the goals touch on professional aspects, and a few representative examples are as follows:

- Establish rapport and maintain a therapeutic relationship with clients of various ages, developmental levels, and cultural backgrounds.
- Assess clients holistically using observation, interview, and evaluation.
- Use clinical reasoning to identify client/patient strengths and needs, and plan appropriate treatment.
- Demonstrate professional behaviors which reflect the profession, and the humanistic values of the larger society.
- Become actively involved in professional organizations on the local, state, and national levels, and participate in community service organizations.

These goals are tied together by themes that run across the curriculum, and include professional behaviors, problem-based learning, clinical reasoning, community service, and both personal and professional growth and development. While this is an OT curriculum, the same ideas and themes would apply equally well to most health care professions.

Program planning parallels can be drawn to the clinical setting since most facilities have a mission statement or philosophy and strategic plan guiding their operation. Individual departments also have stated goals and objectives that relate to the mission of the overall institution. Clinicians are encouraged to contribute to the department and institutional mission; in fact, they are evaluated on their ability to accomplish this. They are also required to be contributing members of a treatment team, and to communicate clearly and concisely both verbally and in writing. To be effective, practitioners must be able to establish rapport, develop, and maintain a therapeutic relationship with clients/patients.

Learning and Teaching Approach

An inquiry and problem-based learning approach is used wherever possible to lay the foundation for critical thinking and clinical reasoning. In fact, the theory course in the spring of the first year incorporates a case study where students are required to integrate and apply theoretical concepts to a hypothetical clinical situation. Activity analysis courses cover media and modalities that are representative and reflective of lifespan activity, and the task analysis process is integrated by applying it to case studies.

Straight lecture is minimized and discussion is maximized to encourage active and participative learning and teaching. Students provide oral presentations on a regular basis, are strongly encouraged to verbally contribute to class, and receive experience and practice in teaching others in labs, lectures, seminars.

Early and frequent self-assessment is used with a measure to look at professional behaviors, and instruments such as the Myers-Briggs Learning Type Indicator. Early and frequent use of the library and the reference desk is encouraged and built into course learning activities. Course objectives are designed to focus on integrating curriculum themes with educational goals and content mastery. Aspects of professional behaviors are integrated and specifically stated in course objectives throughout the curriculum.

The student manual is given to the new class of students during the third class of the introductory course. The session is part of a welcome dinner where the manual is discussed and professional organizations at the national, state, and regional levels are reviewed. The manual incorporates all of the basic information necessary for the new majors; it also includes, among other materials, codes of ethics, standards of practice, regulations, information regarding licensure, and discipline-related terminology. Emphasis is placed on initiating the development of a sense of group solidarity and professional identity. The manual also includes a specific section that presents professional behaviors in considerable detail and discusses their importance and relevance. A number of practical examples of the behaviors in action are provided. Students are required to read the manual and be responsible for the content, and are tested on the material in the introductory course. A student-to-student mentorship program has been developed to facilitate the transition to the university environment and to help with role identity.

Exposure is offered to multiple role models in faculty and community practitioners, who effectively demonstrate professionalism. Extensive use is made of small group activities to increase self-awareness and to enhance the development of professional behaviors. Small, manageable lab sections are scheduled with 12 to 15 students per lab to ensure high quality of learning and teaching experiences.

Clinicians in the practice setting attend and also provide inservice and continuing education experiences. They are required to be active and contributing participants in department and team meetings. Clinicians regu-

larly function in the role of teacher as they provide treatment for clients/patients, and as they instruct families and care givers. A real case study approach to developing practice skills and enhancing professional behaviors can be used by structuring the assignment of a variety of diagnostic categories to broaden clinical experiences. Individual practitioner contribution to departmental objectives can be clarified, and opportunities to contribute to successful outcomes provided.

Evaluation

Students are provided feedback and evaluation on attendance and participation with the goal of facilitating responsible, active, and involved learning. Written and verbal presentation and communication skills are evaluated, and input to guide and encourage growth is given. Case study reports are rated on the criteria of how thoroughly theoretical concepts are integrated and applied to simulated clinical treatment situations.

Summary

The importance and value of the assessment of professional behaviors to health care professions students and practitioners has been demonstrated. Initial reliability and validity information on the *Professional Development Assessment* has been presented. The significance of behaving professionally and ethically to the success and viability of students and clinicians in an ever-changing and dynamic practice environment has been noted.

It is suggested that specific strategies be utilized across curricula and in clinical settings to encourage the development and growth of professional behaviors. The *Professional Development Assessment* can be used on an ongoing basis for self-assessment, as well as developmental and formative evaluation. Ongoing refinement of approaches to enhance professional behaviors must continue in order to develop practitioners who will achieve optimal functioning in today's health care system.

References

Adams, D., Miller, B. K., & Beck, L. (1996). Professional behaviors of hospital nurse executives and middle managers in 10 western states. *Western Journal of Nursing Research, 18(1),* 77-88.

Eddy, D. M., Elfrink, V., Weis, D., & Schank, M. J. (1994). Importance of professional nursing values: A national study of baccalaureate programs. *Journal of Nursing Education, 33,* 257-262.

Gullberg, M. T., Olsson, H. M., Alenfelt, G., Ivarsson, A., &

Nilsson, M. (1994). Ability to solve problems, professionalism, management, empathy, and working capacity in occupational therapy: The professional self-description form. *Scandinavian Journal of Caring Science, 8,* 173- 178.

Kasar, J. (1994). *Enhancing professional behaviors: The Professional Development Assessment.* Paper presented at the Commission on Education, American Occupational Therapy Association annual meeting, Boston, MA.

Kasar, J. (1997). Stability of the Professional Development Assessment. *Perceptual and Motor Skills, 84,* 1373-1374.

Kasar, J., Clark, E. N., Watson, D., & Pfister, S. (1996). *Professional Development Assessment.* Unpublished form.

Kautzmann, L. (1984). *The development of guidelines for feedback on professional behavior in level I fieldwork performance.*

Unpublished doctoral dissertation, Nova University, Milwaukee, WI.

Miller, B. K., Adams, D., & Beck, L. (1993). A behavioral inventory for professionalism in nursing. *Journal of Professional Nursing, 9,* 290-295.

Opacich, K. J., & Hughes, C. J. (1990). *Employer assessment of performance and professional development.* Paper presented at Commission on Education, American Occupational Therapy Association annual meeting, New Orleans, LA.

Thurston, H. I., Flood, M. A., Shupe, I. S., & Gerald, K. B. (1989). Values held by nursing faculty and students in a university setting. *Journal of Professional Nursing, 5,* 199-207.

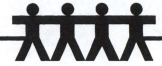

Part Four

Full Circle: Developing Professionalism in the Next Generation

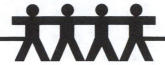

Chapter Fifteen

Learning and Teaching Approaches

Diane E. Watson, MBA, OTR/L, BCP

When students in health care professions become practitioners and move on in their careers to become clinical supervisors and educators, it would generally be agreed that professional education course work and clinical experiences are the primary tools through which individuals: gain the knowledge and skills to practice; acquire the values, principles, and attitudes advocated by a profession; and develop the behaviors required for successful transition to the professional workplace. While there is a body of information regarding the development of cognitive and affective competencies, there are scarce resources to assist in designing learning and teaching approaches that develop or reinforce professional behaviors. Professional behaviors, however, could be considered evidence that individuals possess the knowledge and affective competencies required to be successful in practice. Few would argue that it is within their scope of responsibility to ensure that the conduct of graduates complies with codes of ethics and the professional behaviors expected by society, employers, and peers.

Results of a survey of nursing faculty and students suggests that faculty have significantly higher "essential nursing values" (as measured by the Professional Nursing Behavior Instrument) than baccalaureate students, and teaching experience is positively correlated with value scores (Eddy, Elfrink, Weis, & Schank, 1994). It will be important to determine whether educators are aware of this discrepancy and interested in reducing the disparity between their values and their perceptions of the values held by students. Additionally, if educators' perceptions of student values are based on their observations of student behaviors it would follow that educators would be seeking information and strategies to develop professional behaviors. The growing popularity of seminars on the development and reinforcement of professional behaviors in students probably reflects this need. More research would be required to validate these hypotheses.

This chapter proposes that clinical supervisors and educators, who are interested in developing or reinforcing professional behaviors in students, apply the process that is used to develop and measure students' cognitive and affective competencies, to develop, reinforce, and measure professional behaviors. This process includes the deliberate selection and design of learning objectives, instructional methods, and evaluation instruments. Learning and teaching approaches, however, should parallel the distinctive qualities of different health care professions and educational programs.

The sections and exercises that follow will assist you in defining learning objectives in the domain of professional behaviors and selecting instructional methods that facilitate the development and reinforcement of these behaviors. The objectives and methods chosen by a clinical supervisor or educator, however, must be in congruence with a clinical or educational program's distinctive qualities. A strategy for achieving this congruence will be incorporated into the exercises. Information on the evaluation of professional behaviors after the establishment of learning objectives and selection of instructional methods can be found elsewhere in this text.

Communities, Students, and Professional Education Programs

Professional education programs offer services to meet the evolving needs of their communities and the changing characteristics of their students. These educational services, at a minimum, should enable graduating students to successfully assume a professional career and achieve a sense of personal satisfaction or accomplishment. All professional education programs, however, have distinctive qualities. These distinguishing attributes reflect each program's perceptions of the needs of its community and students, and determination of how these needs should be met. For example, an educational program that is targeted at employed adults in a rural community may use computer technology and distance learning techniques to offer course activities during evening hours. Three distinctive features of this program include the use of computer technology, distance learning techniques, and evening operations.

A program's distinctive qualities are communicated in its mission statement, defined in its curricular goals and objectives, and accomplished through its educational activities. Educational activities are primarily, but not solely, rendered through course work and clinical experiences. Therefore, course and clinical activities should reflect the distinguishing attributes of an educational program, be congruent with the program's curricular goals and objectives, and focus educational efforts. The professional behaviors valued by different programs will likely reflect their distinctive qualities and characteristics. For example, a graduate course for employed professionals may value, define, develop, and reinforce different behaviors than an undergraduate, freshman, entry-level professional program.

cognitive domain (e.g., knowing, comprehending, analyzing, evaluating) and/or in the affective domain (e.g., responding, valuing) (Bloom, Engelhart, Furst, Hill & Krathwohl, 1956; Krathwohl, Bloom & Masia, 1964). Cognitive and affective learning objectives define outcomes in behavioral terms (Bloom et al., 1956; Krathwohl et al., 1964; Mager, 1984). These objectives define expected professional behaviors and provide *observable* and *measurable* evidence that students possess the knowledge, values, and attitudes that an educational program endorses.

Professionals are measured in the workplace on a regular basis. Performance evaluations, peer reviews, quality assurance audits, and client satisfaction questionnaires are examples of instruments that have been designed to measure, monitor, and improve professional conduct. These instruments serve as communication tools to reinforce performance that complies with expectations and highlight discrepancies between current performance and expectations. The domains of performance evaluated on these instruments probably reflect the characteristics and qualities that are valued by particular organizations and service recipients. Continuous assessment of workplace performance reflects society's ongoing need to monitor the knowledge, attitudes, and behaviors of professionals. Learning objectives can provide a proxy for these workplace evaluations by defining expectations and providing a means of measuring the performance of students upon completion of the course or clinical experience.

Learning objectives should reflect the values and principles advocated by the profession, be congruent with the curricular goals and objectives adopted by the educational program, communicate performance expectations, and provide measurable statements about how the instructor expects to observe behavioral change in the desired directions.

Defining Behavioral Expectations and Measuring Performance

The contribution of a specific academic or clinical course to a program's curricular goals and objectives is typically described in the course syllabus and measured with learning objectives. Learning objectives qualify and quantify students' performances upon completion of the course. Change in performance is usually described in the

Congruence with Values and Principles Advocated by the Profession

Designing learning objectives to develop behaviors requires reflection on the values and principles advocated by a particular profession. Code of ethics documents would be useful in this regard. Complete Exercise One by listing the values or principles endorsed by your profession that could potentially be measured by student performance in the course or clinical assignment. Beside the value or principle provide some example behaviors to measure student performance in this domain. For example, the American Occupational Therapy Association (1993) indicates that the seven core attitudes and values that provide the ethical foundation for the profession include altruism, equality, freedom of choice, justice, dignity, truth, and prudence. The nursing profession, physical therapy, and other health care professions have similar values.

Exercise One: Attitudes and Behaviors Advocated by the Profession

Example: *Students will value the inherent worth of each person (i.e., equality and dignity) by listening to and considering the opinions of others.*

1. _____
2. _____
3. _____
4. _____
5. _____

Congruence with Program Mission, Goals, Objectives, and Curriculum Model

Learning objectives should parallel an educational program's mission and contribute to the attainment of curricular goals and objectives. Review the mission statement of your educational institution, college, department, and/or faculty. Identify sentences or phrases that suggest various professional behaviors that are valued by your organization and list these statements in the space provided below. For example, the mission statement of the University of Scranton (1998) in Pennsylvania asserts that the "University understands that ... respect for the dignity and rights of all people must be protected...", "aim of service to the local community...", "excellence in written and oral expression", "reflection on personal experience...".

Exercise Two: Organizational Values

Example: *Students will develop excellence in written and oral expression.*

1. _____
2. _____

3. _____
4. _____
5. _____

Review your program's curricular or clinical department's guiding goals and objectives to identify sentences or phrases that suggest different professional behaviors that are valued. List these statements in the space provided below. Note the program goals that parallel the value statements identified in Exercises One and Two. For example, the goal of the educational program in the Department of Occupational Therapy (1998) at the University of Scranton is to develop graduates who have the "capacity for critical thinking, creative analysis, and clinical reasoning...", "establish rapport...", "a sense of ethical responsibility...", "use their skills and abilities to help others".

Exercise Three: Program Values

Example: *Student will establish and maintain client rapport by valuing the inherent worth, dignity, and rights of each person by responding to the needs and feelings of others, listening to and considering the opinions of others.*

1. _____
2. _____
3. _____
4. _____
5. _____

Communicating Performance Expectations

Learning objectives, in the domain of professional behaviors, should incorporate the value statements and expected behaviors defined in Exercises One through Three, but must communicate performance expectations that are *observable* and *measurable*. Objectives should define and measure changes in student performance, or the outcome or result of instruction; they do not describe the educational process. Explicit objectives communicate to students how to focus and organize their efforts and provide a sound basis for selecting and designing instructional and examination methods (Mager, 1984).

Bloom et al (1956) proposed a popular taxonomy of educational objectives, and provided a structure for the development and measurement of cognitive competencies. The five cognitive components are hierarchically arranged and include knowledge, comprehension, application, analysis or synthesis, and evaluation. Attainment of lower level components such as knowledge occurs before application or evaluation of this information. Krathwohl et al. (1964) extended this taxonomy of educational objectives to address the affective domain by recommending a hierarchy from receiving, to responding, valuing, organizing, and internalizing. Bloom et al. (1956) and Krathwohl et al. (1964) both recommend that educators determine the level of cognitive or affective performance expected and use measurable, behavioral statements of expected outcomes. For example, verbs that illustrate knowledge include define, describe, label, while verbs that illustrate comprehension include explain, paraphrase, and summarize. Learning objectives, in the domain of professional behaviors, should also define in observable and measurable terms the level of competency expected.

Mager (1984) recommends that all instructional objectives include three elements: performance qualities, conditions, and criterion to recognize success. Performance qualities state what the student will be doing when demonstrating mastery of the objective. Behavioral indicators are advocated. Conditions under which these behaviors occur are defined and wherever possible criteria for acceptable performance are also stated. An example objective could be, *"Students will be able to read clinical scenarios and write a progress note, using the problem-oriented medical record format, that includes all relevant client case information."* The performance quality refers to reading clinical information and writing a progress note. The condition implies that students will perform this behavior when provided with written clinical information, and the criterion to recognize success suggests that the note will include relevant information and use a particular format.

Use the recommendations of Bloom et al. (1956), Krathwohl et al. (1964), and Mager (1984) and the information compiled in *Exercise One* through *Exercise Three* to identify and list three professional behaviors that will be developed and measured during your course. One example is provided.

Exercise Four: Professional Behaviors Learning Objectives

Example: *Students will engage in a debate over the relative merits of physical agent modalities versus purposeful activity treatment, verbalize the position of the national association and state licensing board, and listen to the opinions of others.*

1._____

2._____

3._____

Instructional Methods

Once you define course outcome objectives, a determination must be made about the instructional methods that will be employed. This determination defines the process by which change will occur. Students and society as a whole value course work and instruction that is effective and efficient. Course work and instruction are effective when they change students, in desired rather than undesired directions (Mager, 1984); and efficient when this process is conducted with minimal effort, expense, or waste. Given the limited availability of research literature on the relative effectiveness of different instructional formats in developing professional behaviors, Table 15-1 reviews the scope of instructional methods used by educators in light of intent to develop professional behaviors. This table provides a summary of the potential utility of various learning and teaching methods to develop or reinforce the professional behaviors delineated on the *Professional Development Assessment* (Kasar, Clark, Watson, & Pfister, 1996). You are also encouraged to review the Additional Resources section of this chapter for more information.

Summary

The workplace conduct and performance of professional practitioners is monitored and evaluated, and so should the development of professional behaviors in students and beginning clinicians. This chapter proposes that educators and clinical supervisors begin the process by explicitly defining expected behaviors in course and program learning objectives, and selecting instructional methods to achieve these results. Research is limited, however, on the cost effectiveness of different instructional strategies on developing professional behaviors. Although this chapter presents an array of methods that have been proposed in the area of health care professions and services, many of the suggestions are appropriate to educators in other fields. In addition, the authors of many other chapters in this text have proposed learning and teaching approaches that can be used by students, clinicians, and educators.

Table 15-1

LEARNING AND TEACHING APPROACHES FOR VARIOUS PROFESSIONAL BEHAVIORS IN THE HEALTH CARE PROFESSIONS*

Professional Behavior	Learning and Teaching Approaches
Dependability	Classroom clinics. Clinic visits. Community outings. Community service initiatives. Debate teams. Faculty assistantships. Group projects. Practitioner mentors. Role models. Student involvement in writing and research activities of faculty.
Professional Presentation	Classroom clinics. Clinic visits. Community outings. Community service initiatives. Interdisciplinary projects. Interviewing potential clients or other professionals. Lab activities, projects, and assignments. Faculty assistantships. Marketing projects. Practitioner mentors. Project leaders—elected or appointed. Role models. Student portfolio or vitae of accomplishments. Student directed research. Student involvement in writing and research activities of faculty. Verbal defense of position papers.
Initiative	Choice of assignments. Community service initiatives. Faculty assistantships. Interviewing individuals with disabilities in the community, potential client agencies, or other health service professionals. Self-selecting a practitioner mentor from a roster. Role models. Self-selected projects. Student involvement in writing and research activities of faculty. Student portfolio or vitae of accomplishments. Student directed research.
Empathy	Community service initiatives. Cross cultural exercises or experiences. Group projects. Peer reviews. Reading about disability experiences. Role models. Watching videos about disability experiences. Writing client narratives. Writing journals or diaries.
Cooperation	Debate teams. Faculty assistantships. Group projects. Interdisciplinary projects. Lab activities, projects, and assignments. Project leaders—elected or appointed. Role models. Student involvement in writing and research activities of faculty.
Organization	Community service initiatives. Complex assignments with short deadlines. Faculty assistantships. Role models. Student associations, societies, or ad hoc committees. Student directed research. Student involvement in writing and research activities of faculty. Student sponsored symposiums.
Clinical Reasoning	Case method. Classroom clinics. Debate teams. Internship experiences. Lab activities, projects, and assignments. Role models. Student directed research. Student involvement in writing and research activities of faculty. Writing client narratives.
Supervisory Process	Juried poster presentations. Juried publication of student papers or research. Peer reviews and feedback—anonymous, formative, summative, written, and/or verbal. Project leaders—elected or appointed.
Verbal Communication	Community service initiatives. Debates. Faculty assistantships. Interdisciplinary and multidisciplinary projects. Marketing projects. Practitioner mentors. Peer reviews. Role models. Simulated case conferences. Student involvement in writing and research activities of faculty. Student lecture presentations. Verbal defense of position paper. Verbal class participation.
Written Communication	Marketing projects. Peer reviews. Poster presentations. Refereed student paper publications. Student portfolio or vitae of accomplishments. Student directed research. Student involvement in writing and research activities of faculty. Written assignments, essays, and client narratives. Written case histories.

*Instructional methods are listed alphabetically, not on the basis of effectiveness.

Attainment of performance targets will require continuous formative feedback to students, which can be provided by peers, colleagues, mentors, and educators. Summative evaluation must also parallel the expectations that have been specified in the cognitive, affective, and professional behavior domains. Information on summative evaluation is discussed in the previous chapter on the assessment of professional behaviors.

References

Bloom, B. S., Engelhart, M. D., Furst, E. J., Hill, W.H., & Krathwohl, D.R. (1956). *Taxonomy of educational objectives: The classification of educational goals. Handbook 1: Cognitive domain.* New York, NY: Longman.

Department of Occupational Therapy, University of Scranton. (1998). *1997/1998 Student manual.* Scranton, PA: University of Scranton Press.

Eddy, D. M., Elfrink, V., Weis, D., & Schank, M. J. (1994). Importance of professional nursing values: A national study of baccalaureate programs. *Journal of Nursing Education, 33,* 257-262.

Kasar, J., Clark, E. N., Watson, D., & Pfister, S. (1996) *Professional development assessment.* Unpublished form.

Krathwohl, D. R., Bloom, B. S., & Masia, B. B. (1964). *Taxonomy of educational objectives: The classification of educational goals. Handbook II: Affective domain.* New York, NY: Longman.

Mager, R. F. (1984). *Measuring instructional results: Got a match?* Belmont, CA: Pitman Learning.

Mager, R. F. (1984). *Preparing instructional objectives,* 2nd Edition. Belmont, CA: Pitman Learning.

University of Scranton. (1998). *1997/1998 Undergraduate student catalogue.* Scranton, PA: University of Scranton Press.

Additional Resources

Bechtel N. (1993). Commentary on incompetent, unethical, or illegal practice — teaching students to cope. *ENA's Nursing Scan in Emergency Care, 3(6),* 18.

Brookfield, S. D. (1988). *Developing critical thinkers: Challenging adults to explore alternative ways of thinking and acting.* San Francisco, CA: Jossey-Bass.

Gronlund, N. E. (1978). *Stating objectives for classroom instruction.* New York, NY: MacMillan.

Harrow, A. J. (1972). *A taxonomy of the psychomotor domain.* New York, NY: Longman.

Neistadt, M. E. (1996). Teaching strategies for the development of clinical reasoning. *American Journal of Occupational Therapy, 50,* 676-684.

Peloquin, S. M. (1996). Art: An occupation with promise for developing empathy. *American Journal of Occupational Therapy, 50,* 655-661.

Sviden, G., & Saljo, R. (1993). Perceiving patients and their nonverbal reactions. *American Journal of Occupational Therapy, 47,* 491-497.

Young-Mason, J. (1988). Literature as a mirror to compassion ... to study the implications of moral behavior... Sophocles' philoctetes. *Journal of Professional Nursing, 4,* 299-301.

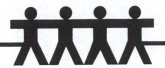

Chapter Sixteen

Continuing Education

Paul Petersen, PhD, OTR/L

Background

Between graduation and advanced practice lie the novice and apprentice years when new graduates emerge from their lack of confidence and develop into master clinicians. While many factors contribute to this process, continuing education (CE) is in the forefront.

One Issue is Confidence

Students often enter their clinical assignments and subsequent careers with limited confidence in their knowledge and skills. This is to be expected. A lot of what was learned up until now remains "head knowledge", until reinforced in a variety of situations. Students of one program may compare their education with others from different schools, and ask "Why didn't they teach me that?" Do not fall into this trap. The area of content emphasized varies from one college/university program to another. Different frames of reference and approaches from an array of schools add a certain richness to any profession.

Just the Basics

Any medical or health care professions educator will admit that what is covered in school are just the basics, and that this is bolstered somewhat with the clinical education that is integrated with and follows academic preparation. Faculty will also admit, unfortunately, that new

information is advancing at such a rate that what is learned today will be out of date in a few years, if that long.

As a soon-to-be provider, accept the fact that what you learn in school will not be enough for the years to come, but it is more than sufficient for the time being. As an accredited program, your curriculum has been through numerous reviews at the departmental and university levels. It also has undergone strict review by an outside professional accreditation agency. The important point is to learn and apply your school's curriculum content to the best of your ability. As you gain confidence, you will find new areas of application, and through this process, your base of knowledge will grow.

Learning Styles

It should be remembered that various professions have differing perspectives, approaches, and historical evolutions and underpinnings. Some emphasize technology, while others may have a greater call for manual dexterity and/or verbal skill. Our learning styles vary with the person and/or the knowledge base of the profession. Some can gain all they need to keep up to date through the computer database and review articles. Others may do better with a presentation and hands-on demonstration. Professional organizations, journal clubs, graduate courses, study groups, lunchtime inservice programs, and informal information exchange and networking all serve to keep us current.

The Need for Continuing Education

The chapters in this text have addressed the components of professionalism not typically covered in courses such as physiology, child development, orthopedic assessment, and wound care. The argument has been made that behaviors such as empathy (Chapter 7) and cooperation (Chapter 8), for example, significantly augment the knowledge base of a successful provider. In Chapter 4, dependability was emphasized in the call from patients for their practitioners to be knowledgeable and up to date in their fields. When professionals do not keep up in their specialty areas, patients see them as undependable, and trust can be weakened or broken. State licensure and professional certification may require providers to exhibit continued competence, often through attendance and participation in CE.

The Growing Pace of Knowledge

Keeping up to date is surprisingly difficult given today's push for production and generation of institutional income. The number of health care-related journals, including some emphasizing research, has grown tremendously. Computerization has facilitated database production and retrieval that allows for compilation of vast statistics which link findings from around the world. The acquisition of this information is becoming easier and cheaper to find through the various web sites for both the professional and layman. For example, one prime time television show featured a junior high student who diagnosed his own cancer on a school computer network. Technology is out there, and research is increasing a health care profession's body of knowledge on an ongoing basis. The issue is how to compile all this into a workable, manageable, and reviewable format of theory and application for the busy clinician.

Professional Requirements

While I am encouraging you to pursue continuing eduction opportunities, this may not be an option; it may be mandatory if you want to continue to practice. The issue is highly variable and differs from state to state and profession to profession. It's up to you to scrutinize the requirements of your professional accrediting body (ANA, ASHA, AMA, APTA, AOTA, etc.) and your state regulatory or licensing agency. Issues in CE and compe-tency have received considerable attention, and new resolutions and mandates are appearing on a regular basis. Change is as rapid as that found in health care reform. The important point to know is that your profession, area of practice, and geographical location influence your requirements, so you should be current on the regulations specific to you. This is especially important if you have a travelling position which takes you from state to state every several months.

Continuing Education

Purpose

The purpose of CE is to offer pertinent theoretical, clinical, and/or practical content to health care professionals in a convenient but intense and focused format. There are also courses in administration, publishing, teaching, grant writing, supervision, and more. The content of each course is narrowly focused on a given topic, and varies from basic to advanced levels of expected audience expertise. Levels of the course are specified, in advance, through the course and conference brochures. The most common format is an intense weekend course, but length may range from a half-day seminar to a 2-week course. Instruction by nationally known speakers who tour from city to city across the country is typically advertised in metropolitan areas. Universities and medical centers may sponsor regional workshops. Courses which concentrate on a specialty certification may require some '"homework" following the session, or between part one and part two of a series of courses. This may include written papers and reports, testing, case studies, clinical trials, and others.

Health care providers take advantage of CE to refresh themselves on a given topic, learn a new body of knowledge, obtain a specialty certification (e.g., cardiac care), and/or address requirements of their state or professional organizations. Update and retooling courses are one means of re-entry to the profession after years of absence. They include an overview of basic professional competencies and are specific to a given profession.

A relatively new format is known as the pre-conference institute. These are half-day to 2-day long CE events attached to the beginning or end of a state or national convention. Another recent format is the CE correspondence course where credit is obtained through home study, usually sanctioned through one's professional society, and most recently workshops are being offered by teleconferencing. The next steps are distance learning and videoconferencing.

Identifying Courses

No matter where your interests lie, the wide world of CE is ready to serve you. Identifying availability of upcoming courses is relatively easy. The information literally comes to you! Once you are licensed, certified, and/or registered, your name will appear on numerous mailing lists. My mailbox often overflows with course brochures, and my journals are replete with advertisements. As some of my interests are interdisciplinary, I check the bulletin boards and weekly publications of other professions to see what is offered that may be of interest to me. What is more important than finding a course is finding a "good" course. There are often many courses on a given topic, so careful selection is important. It is often more valid to select a course based on the speaker than on a close geographical proximity. A short drive and the cost of a hotel room are well worth it to sit under the tutelage of a nationally recognized authority.

Call Ahead for Details

If there is ever a question on a course, feel free to call the sponsoring organization or presenter for details. CE courses are generally expensive, and you do not want to waste your money on an ill-suited one. Over my career, almost all of the courses I attended have been beneficial. In only one instance did I leave a course early, but I have been in workshops where a participant was very dissatisfied. This was not related to the quality of the course; the course was just not what that person thought it would be. Either the course brochure was unclear or the participant did not read it thoroughly.

Course Level

You should also verify the content level of the course. There is nothing worse than being in an advanced course when you are just starting out, and all that is presented is going over your head. This is just as true for an experienced professional finding him- or herself in a novice workshop. After registering for a CE course, a former colleague was called by a presenter who wanted to explain the course, and see if it was what she really was looking for. My colleague was from a different profession, and the presenter just wanted to be sure that the match was right. The course turned out to be a wonderful experience.

CE courses typically focus on a specific area of practice and theory. Presentation format may vary in combinations of lecture, patient demonstration, lab practice, role play, and question-and-answer sessions. Audiovisuals play a significant role in the learning and teaching process. Handouts, outlines, and author reprints often augment the topic.

Additional Benefits

In addition to gaining a body of knowledge in a compact, compressed, and time-efficient manner, there are side benefits to attending CE sessions. Many participants are very knowledgeable in their field, some being on the cutting edge. Over the years, I have been most impressed with the participants I have met while taking CE courses. The opportunities to share with others are plentiful.

Networking is continual and ongoing, and I know that course participation has resulted in finding employment, identifying staff, locating collaborators for a research project, and much more. Through informal discussion you can find out about additional CE courses in your area of interest, especially to determine or identify which are the good ones and which are not. Given the chance, CE at distant sites is a great opportunity to just get away, visit old friends in the evening, or see the sights. While the main purpose is to learn, some rest and relaxation is good for the "professional soul".

Who Pays for Continuing Education?

Prior to health care reform, institutions were more liberal with financial support for CE courses. As a former university instructor, I often encouraged students to ask for a "start-up" CE course as part of a hiring package. This is rarely the case anymore. The dollars are tight, and time away from the clinic is lost revenue in a very cost-conscious and competitive market. However, funding has not dried up completely, otherwise there would be no market for CE. Needless to say, funding is available; it is just not as easy to come by as before.

It is true that some facilities are in a position to remain generous with support while others have set up strict guidelines. Some new hires may have to serve on staff for a few years before they are eligible to apply for a course. Other places may require a formal proposal, including a description of financial benefits to the organization. Smart managers know that very specialized education may serve as the basis for a new product or program, and thus, additional income. It would benefit a staff member to do some research as to needs for a new program and consider a proposal. This may develop into additional courses, staff, and equipment while the institution ultimately derives the financial benefits.

In the United States we have come to expect that someone else will pay for whatever is good for us. Take health care, for example. In the past, most individuals paid for their health care up until the 1950s. Then, two things happened. Health insurance blossomed and some employers attached payment for health care as a side benefit to get good workers. Now we just expect these benefits. We view it as a right. The rest is history. Technology arrived, and we live much longer. There have been both abuse of the reimbursement system and inflation of medical care costs. Malpractice litigation has become an industry. And now we are seeing that some people are again paying for their health care or parts of it. There is nothing wrong with this, and people maintain the ability to choose. The reason that I am bringing this up is that there is no reason that we cannot pay for our own CE, at least once in a while. If we know that there is additional information and material necessary to keep on top of things in our practice, we should do whatever it takes to acquire this new or updated information.

Alternative Continuing Education

There are some less traditional alternatives in CE. Some facilities will hire a well-known speaker to come in and teach a topic needed by their staff members. They use their own clinics and auditorium on a weekend, and open the course up to some others in the community to attend for a fee. This way they get the training less expensively or may even make a modest profit, and the institution provides an important community service to local professionals.

Exchange of services is an additional method to consider. There are many ways to do this. In a health care alliance, for example, staff members can do some "on-the-job training" for a week at a sister institution elsewhere in the region. They can work side-by-side with those having the expertise. The personal network is another possibility. Many of the health care professions are relatively small,

and members often have contacts across the country. Using the informal network, a supervisor contacts a colleague with expertise in a given area and asks if a staff member can go and observe at his or her facility for a few days or a week. All that may be involved are travel and housing costs.

Continuing Education Credit and Transfer

All CE courses provide CE credit for their participants. This is necessary for those with professional requirements to regularly attend a minimum amount of CE. You will receive a certificate of participation at the end of the course signed by the sponsor and/or speaker which lists the date(s), contact hours, and title. Do not lose this proof of attendance. Make a photocopy for your files at work and give one to your supervisor. Be sure to check the annual or biannual requirements for the organization that issues your license or specialty certification. How many credits do they require each year?

The basic credit unit is the *contact hour*. In this method, a day and a half long course providing 12 classroom hours of instruction earns the participant 12 contact hours. Sometimes they are referred to as *credit hours*. Another method to quantify attendance is the CEU or CE unit. This is calculated by dividing the contact hours by 10. Thus, if you attend an 11-hour course, you receive 11 contact or credit hours and 1.1 CEU.

The regulatory agencies of several states require that CE courses offered in their states for credit must be approved by the agencies in advance. This has caused a nightmare in paperwork and bureaucracy for the sponsoring agencies and participants. Be sure to find out in advance if the course you attend will be accepted by your state agency. Whenever you have questions, call the course sponsor and/or regulatory or credentialing agency.

Choosing a CE Course

Deciding what CE course to take may be complex. There are multiple influences to consider. Sometimes the choice is easy. Your supervisor sends you to attend such and such a course to benefit you and your department. Other times the choice is yours. Certainly course tuition, location, distance, travel, and housing expenses must be factored in.

The best way to choose a course or a sequence of courses is to first develop a long-range plan for yourself. Most new clinicians change jobs frequently as their professional career plans evolve. Ask yourself the following: What are your short-term and long-term goals? Where do you see yourself in a year, in 5 years, in 10? Do you want to remain in clinical practice? Do you eventually see yourself as an administrator, faculty member, researcher? Do you like to present topics yourself, to write and publish? How about grant writing? Would you like to be a master clinician? Do you plan to stay in health care? How do your goals match with program needs? While career development is beyond the scope of this chapter, it is important to realize that CE will be an important component in your future. It will be more meaningful when you have a definite plan of action based on direction from some good mentors.

Before You Leave

The remainder of this chapter will address recommendations pertinent to the CE process itself. This includes tips for before, during, and after the course.

A Staff Inservice Presentation

The purpose of this section is to help you optimize your CE experience. Here are some recommendations to consider prior to your departure for the course. One of the best ways to learn new material is to teach it to peers. Before you go, arrange with your supervisor or departmental inservice coordinator to conduct a lunchtime presentation for the staff after the course. Set a date and time! Give yourself some space, as it will take time for you to condense the material from a weekend course into a meaningful hour-long session. The time interval will allow you to review and apply what you have learned to further reinforce what you share with others. If you wait too long, however, you might misplace your course handouts and get tied up in the daily routine, thus losing the spark that follows a good course.

The Physical Environment

Prepare for the environment of the CE classroom. Many courses are held in hotels—not the most suitable place for learning, but they are conveniently located, often near airports. When this occurs, the sponsoring organization and/or presenters are not always familiar with the physical surroundings, particularly the lighting

and temperature control. The room may be too warm or too cool, so dress accordingly so that you can take off a layer or add a layer to be comfortable. The weekend staff from the hotel may able to correct the situation, but it could take some time. In the middle of my presentation at a state convention one fall, two participants got up, stating as they left the room, "Nothing personal with what you are saying, but it's freezing in here." Some others nodded in agreement, but remained.

Along with possible temperature problems are lighting limitations. Most speakers use audiovisuals, requiring that the lights be dimmed. Sometimes it is not possible to dim the lights; it is all or nothing. You can't write in the dark. So, to take notes, bring a small flashlight. In fact, I once had to loan my light to the speaker who could not see his notes on the podium once the lights went out, and the slides were an important component of his presentation. Another variation is a pen made for writing at night with a light built into it. I once observed a participant using a pen to take notes, and she had a mini flashlight attached to the pen providing just the light necessary to write. Like the temperature, hotel lighting is complex, so it may not always be possible to correct the problem immediately.

More on Clothing

For clinical courses in PT and OT, for example, lab clothes are often required. Wear what you think will be comfortable if you will have your shoulder, lower extremity, and/or lumbar spine evaluated.

Seating

Seating can be anything from metal folding chairs to plush theater seats, and you may be sitting for several hours at a time. If you suffer from back trouble, consider bringing your back support cushion along or a small seat cushion if hard chairs are a hardship to you.

Some Items to Take with You

Besides the flashlight, there are some other items that I recommend you take along. If you do not need them, that is fine, but you may wish you had them. As stated earlier, CE is an expensive investment, so take some steps in advance to reduce the risk of any irritating and nagging problems that hinder your learning. Bring a pad of paper, clipboard, and a writing instrument. Sounds basic, but not all conferences supply these. There may be no space in the handouts to scribble notes, or the little hotel note pad that is supplied may be insufficient to meet your needs. They were meant for recording messages by the telephone, and not all facilities supply pens. The clipboard is useful if there is no table on which to write. There may only be chairs. Or you may wish to take notes while lying or sitting on the floor. If your course has a lab component there is often considerable movement to the front of the room to observe a demonstration. It is not easy to take notes as part of a large group if participants are crowding around a small demonstration table. The clipboard makes note-taking easy and your notes will be easier to read a week later.

Bring a few colored markers or a four-color pen to highlight your note-taking, especially if anatomy will be addressed. Every time I learned neuroanatomy we copied the alpha motor neurons in red and the gammas in green. A transparent highlighter is very useful to accentuate special texts or sections from both your notes and the conference handouts. I was always glad I did this when reviewing my materials later on. Speaking of anatomy, take along a small anatomy text or make a copy of a page or two of pertinent subject matter for quick reference. If your course is on swallowing disorders, for example, a copy of the head and neck anatomy may be most useful. Finally, if you or your department owns the text authored by the course speaker, bring it along to be autographed. It will make a nice addition to your library.

If you are going to a course covering a body of knowledge with which you have some experience, take some time before you leave to compile a list of questions for the speaker. This is a good time to get some answers on further theory development, latest research, or a difficult patient you are treating.

The Basics: Water, Food, and Air

For your personal comfort, carry a refillable bottle of water to the course. Many hotels provide glasses and water pitchers on the table, but you cannot count on this in advance. A water fountain may be available, but it is a long time between breaks. The environment is usually dry, and the air is recirculated in the often windowless conference or ballrooms. Tuck a package of mints into your carryall. Use your breaks to get outside whenever possible for fresh air.

A benefit to many attending an out of town CE course is the opportunity to enjoy a good meal out. This may be fine once a day, but hotel meals are very expensive and may provide more food than you need, especially if you sit most of the day. Because of this I always take along fruit and bread products that remain fresh for several days for lunches or breaks. In addition, I carry some tea bags and coffee packets should these not be available during the breaks.

Your Travel Checklist

A good friend of mine was a full-time CE director for many years at a teaching medical center in the Midwest. At conference time she went out of her way to help the participants with items they forgot, the most common being their glasses or a container of prescription medication. There were many other items. For any travel you undertake, whether it be for CE or vacation, it is a good idea to compile a checklist in advance containing items to bring. Maintain the list over the years, and experience will help you refine it so that you take along only what is necessary. If you are flying to your destination, always pack light. Don't forget some extra business cards for networking purposes. At the end of the checklist give yourself a reminder to leave a phone number, and if possible, a contact person so that you can be reached by your family in an emergency, day and night. Someone back home may need this information.

During the Course

A Thorough Set of Notes

There are a few things to do during the course to improve your retention of the topic. CE is very intense, and you will not come away mastering all the information presented. Mastery will require your time and review in the weeks and months following your return. The course will only be as good as your memory and your notes. I sometimes have 30 to 40 pages of handwritten notes from a 2 to 3 day course. During the course, insure that your notes are as complete as possible to serve you at a later date. You will need to rely on your handwritten notes and handouts as your link to the course that is now long over. I recommend that you ask the speakers for any clarification on the content in their handouts. If an issue is not clear now, it will be even less meaningful in the weeks to come.

Ask Questions

Take the first 5 minutes of each break and review your notes for thoroughness. Presenters speak fast, and an important slide may only be on the screen briefly. If there are gaps in your notes, find out now and talk to the speaker. Then at the end of each day, read over your notes, use your highlighter, and do a second check for gaps or areas in need of clarification. Usually the first few minutes of the day are to answer questions from the materials presented the day before. This review session is only valuable if you go prepared and have questions ready to ask. Once you are home, review your notes every month or so, and you will be surprised how items which were previously of little application will now pop out at you.

Note Complete Citations for Easy Retrieval

If the speaker refers to important references in the bibliography, be sure that the citation is complete with date, source, and pages. It might be difficult to obtain a copy of a particular article. If you would eventually like a copy of a certain reference, make a notation on the bibliography to remind you after you are home. Your institution's interlibrary loan program should be able to locate any source for you. Don't rely on your memory. After a short time interval, you may not remember which references are the ones of importance.

Personalize Your Notes

If a large part of your practice is clinical, the following tip will be valuable. Many CE courses are clinically oriented and present many new methods of evaluation and patient care. Recently I have attended several of these valuable courses, and patients whom I was treating at that time came to mind. So I jotted down their names in the margin of my notes or course outline near the procedure that applied to them. Once I returned, I was able to sift through the margins of my notes and locate these reminders; for example, a new way to test Mr. Jones, or an item of patient education related to her situation to share with Mrs. Smith.

Are Any Handouts Missing?

Finally, let me offer two more quick items pertaining to the handouts. First, print your name on the cover or folder immediately. In a room of 40-plus people with purple binders, it is easy to confuse ownership. With your name on it, there will be no question which one is yours when you return from a break. Second, review your notes to make sure all the materials are there. Collating errors can happen, and if you do not notice that something is missing now, it will be missing forever. Not all speakers follow their handouts, but issue them for your later reference. If you are uncertain whether anything is missing, compare your set of handouts against that of another participant.

Check Your Tables

This last bit of advice addresses CE courses with patient demonstration and practice labs. If the course is in a hotel with hotel conference tables or a clinic with lightweight portable examination tables brought in for the occasion, check underneath yours before you or your partner lie or sit on it. If you change tables, check again. This is to be sure that the mechanisms which lock the table legs are in place. Conduct your check every time you change tables and every morning of the course, as they may be removed and returned overnight to accommodate other hotel activities. I have seen problems several times — a participant is lying supine on the table and the head or foot end of it collapses. Injuries can result.

Course Feedback

Near the end of the course you will be asked to complete a feedback sheet regarding the speaker(s), program, facilities, etc. While you are usually in a rush to get home, try to take a few minutes to offer meaningful feedback. Sponsoring agencies take your input very seriously and adjust their courses accordingly. While often thought of as complaint sheets, these forms offer the opportunity to state what was special about this course and offer constructive criticism in detail. Be sure to mention what you liked best along with your helpful suggestions for improvements.

After You Return

Many of the recommendations for this section have already been mentioned. This includes following through with a short inservice for your staff and reviewing your notes and handouts routinely upon your return. As you proceed in clinical practice, add clinical findings to your CE notes, and include additional references you may identify. I suggest that unless you had ample practice during the course with a new procedure, you first try it out on a spouse or colleague before using it with a patient. My son has been my willing guinea pig over the years.

If your speakers leave you a phone number to call them with questions following the course, they mean for you to do this. I have both called speakers and received calls from former participants of courses I taught. In every case, the exchange was meaningful and cordial.

Graduate Education

CE is one means of acquiring additional knowledge, and it meets the needs of many practicing clinicians as they develop and refine their skills. It is not, however, the only way toward professional development. CE has its limitations. A major drawback is that it may be piecemeal. The knowledge you obtain through a selection of CE courses may lack the depth or breadth you need. Graduate education is an alternative. The commitment will be greater but so will the rewards. There may be flexibility in funding such a program and adjusting your work schedule around your studies, whether full or part-time.

Conclusion

This chapter has described CE in detail. I hope I have conveyed the importance of this form of education both to maintain and accelerate your professional career after graduation. You may be bound by regulation and certification requirements to pursue CE, but it is more important that you recognize its value and pursue it on your own, regardless of the requirements. You owe this much to your patients. There are additional benefits to course attendance through subsequent relationships and networking with fellow course participants.

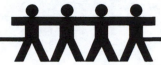

Part Five

Reality Rehearsal: Structured Activities for Professional Behaviors©

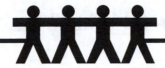

Structured Activity #1

Be Careful What You Write©

Jack Kasar,
PhD, OTR/L

E. Nelson Clark,
MS, OTR/L

Be Careful What You Write

Goal

Emphasize the importance of communication skills in writing and interpreting written instructions.

Objectives

Participants will describe a complicated procedure, in writing, to be performed by another participant in order to:
- Communicate to other participants in writing.
- Interpret another participant's written communication.
- Discuss the importance of communicating ideas clearly and concisely in writing.
- Demonstrate analyzing, synthesizing, and interpreting written information.
- Demonstrate an inquiring or questioning approach in writing.

Group Size

Unlimited. Space to write and carry out exercise must be available. Supplies must be available to all participants.

Time Frame

Fifteen minutes to synthesize and write. Fifteen minutes to follow instructions and write inquiries if needed. Thirty minutes discussion.

Materials Needed

- Pen only. (Sorry...no pencils please)
- 8 1/2 by 11 copier or printer paper
- Clothespins. Wire spring type with 2 wooden pieces. Enough for 1/2 of the number of participants.
- Mousetraps. Wooden platform type with spring loaded wire trap (the old fashioned kind). Enough for 1/2 the number of participants.

Process

MOUSETRAP!

1) The instructor divides the group in half, assigns each member a partner, and dismisses one of the halves to wait in another area so the two halves are not aware of each other.
2) The instructor distributes mousetrap, paper, and pen to the half (Group #1) remaining in the room.
3) Group #1 is instructed to: "write a step by step procedure for setting the mousetrap." A small paper ball (dare say a "spitball"?) may be used for the "cheese" to bait the trap. This group has 15 minutes to accomplish this task.
4) At the close of 15 minutes, invite Group #2 back into the room and reunite with assigned partner.
5) Instruct both groups that there are to be *no* verbal interactions until the exercise is completed (at the end of the additional 15 minutes).

© J. Kasar and N. Clark 1998

6) Instruct Group #2 to use the written instructions "Only" to set and bait the mousetraps. "No fair using previous experience"!

7) If questions or inquiries are needed from a member of Group #2 to accomplish the task, they must make a written inquiry to their partner in Group #1. The Group #1 member must respond in writing.

8) Watch those fingers!

Remember, participation is voluntary and individuals should feel free to not participate if they are uncomfortable with the activity.

CLOTHESPIN (ADDITIONAL ACTIVITY)

1) Switch groups. Send Group #1 outside for this exercise.

2) Instruct Group #2 to disassemble the clothespin and write instructions for reassembling the clothespin.

3) Invite Group #1 back into the room (Remember, *no* talking).

4) Have the partner in Group #1 reassemble the clothespin from Group #2 partner's instructions. Same communication rules apply as in the mousetrap exercise.

5) Instructor leads group discussion on:

    a) Humorous occurrences in group

    b) Problems encountered

    c) Actual health care problems related to writing and communications, such as recent news occurrences where a health care worker makes a serious mistake because of inaccurate written communication.

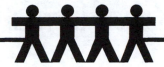

Structured
Activity #2

Judging Books by
Their Cover©

Jack Kasar,
PhD, OTR/L

E. Nelson Clark,
MS, OTR/L

Judging Books by Their Cover

Goal

Participants will increase awareness of one's professional demeanor by evaluating other participants on how they look and behave.

Objectives

- Judge other participants on their appearance/behaviors
- Discuss how individuals want others to perceive them
- Discuss the importance of body posture/language
- Discuss how previous values and attitudes have an effect on becoming a professional

Group Size

Unlimited. Space must be available for participants to move about and observe others or observe from a group circle formation.

Time Frame

Thirty minutes to observe, thirty minutes of discussion.

Materials Needed

- "Judging A Book By the Cover" worksheet
- Pen/pencil

Process

1) The instructor distributes worksheets.
2) Participants instructed to look about the room, observe other participants. Participants may walk about but refrain from talking.
3) Participants encouraged to observe body language, clothing, hairstyles, or any feature that would form an opinion.
4) Participants encouraged to make note of a previous event in their life that caused them to formulate a certain opinion/judgement/belief about the participant they are observing.
5) After 30 minutes observing time, instructor begins to encourage participants to disclose their observations and the reasons for their observations/opinions.
6) The worksheets have been constructed to elicit positive characteristics. However, the instructor should be sensitive to certain observations that may emerge and be prepared to handle comments that some of the participants may find discouraging/offensive.

Judging a Book by the Cover

1. Find someone who looks like they enjoy children.
   Reason:

2. Find someone who looks like they play sports.
   Reason:

3. Find an animal lover. One who takes care of and raises animals.
   Reason:

4. Find a person who looks ambitious. One who gets the job done.
   Reason:

5. Find one who appreciates classical music.
   Reason:

6. Find the one who likes modern rock and roll music.
   Reason:

7. Find someone who looks daring and would appreciate exciting activities.
   Reason:

8. Find an interesting conversationalist. Someone you could listen to.
   Reason:

9. Find a gourmet cook or one who would enjoy gourmet cooking.
   Reason:

10. Find a sophisticated looking person. Go for the refined look.
    Reason:

11. Who looks intelligent in this group (you cannot list yourself).
    Reason:

Structured Activity #3

Build a Better Mousetrap©

Jack Kasar,
PhD, OTR/L

E. Nelson Clark,
MS, OTR/L

Build a Better Mousetrap

Goal

Emphasize the importance of cooperation and the skills involved in working effectively in a group.

Objectives

Participants will engage in a small group activity of building a "mousetrap" in order to:
- Examine their role in a small group task
- Identify key behaviors that contributed positively to the group
- Develop an awareness of another's behavior and the result of those behaviors

Group Size

Five or six individuals comprise each group. Space to work on a small table top. Space to write and complete exercise must be available.

Time Frame

Twenty minutes to complete task, fifteen minutes to complete written portion of task, thirty minutes discussion.

Materials Needed

- Styrofoam blocks (3 each, 6" x 6")
- Clay (1 tennis ball size)
- Construction paper (3 full sheets)
- Pipe cleaners (6 each)

- String (3 ft)
- Small brads/finishing nails (12)
- Scissors (1 pair)
- Blunt modeling knife

Process

1) The instructor divides the group into small groups of five or six members.
2) The instructor gives each group a set of the above listed materials.
3) The group is instructed as follows: "As a group, I would like for you to use the tools and materials provided to build a better mousetrap. You have 15 minutes to accomplish this task." "Questions?" The instructor may only repeat the initial instructions. "Begin the group".
4) During the group's construction phase, the instructor will want to observe key negative behaviors such as, refusal to participate (withdrawal), dictatorship, excessive clowning, etc. Key positive behaviors should also be noted such as rewarding comments (praises), supportive encouragement, and productive active involvement.
5) At the 20 minute period, call time. Ask the group to elect a member to describe the mousetrap to the other groups.
6) Give supportive and positive comments to all of the groups for accomplishing the task.

7) On an individual piece of paper for each group, have the group answer the following questions:

   a) Was there too much or too little time to accomplish the task?

   b) Were there any unclear directions or concepts associated with this project? If so explain.

   c) Identify each member's contribution to the project, i.e., what did they make or say to help the project.

   d) Identify positive behaviors (specific examples) exhibited by members of the group that made the other members feel good about their participation.

   e) What was the result of this positive interaction.

   f) Identify problem-solving techniques or communication techniques used to accomplish this task.

   g) Identify events, positive or negative, that influenced the task outcome.

Structured Activity #4

Being on Time©

Jack Kasar,
PhD, OTR/L

E. Nelson Clark,
MS, OTR/L

Being on Time

Goal

Emphasize the importance of "being on time".

Objectives

Participants will complete the questionnaire worksheet and participate in group discussion in order to:
• Define "being on time".
• Elaborate on the importance of "being on time".
• Relate incidents (1 humorous and 1 serious) about "not" being on time.
• Identify places or events where it is difficult to be "on time".
• Identify reasons that cause you to be "late".
• Explore mechanisms that will assist in "being on time".

Group Size

Unlimited. Space to write and complete worksheet.

Time Frame

Fifteen minutes to synthesize and write. Thirty minutes discussion and story sharing.

Materials Needed

• Worksheet
• Pencil

Being On Time

What does "being on time" mean to you:

Explain the importance that "being on time" has in your life, i.e., what could be consequences?

Relate two incidents, one humorous and one serious, caused by you not being on time.

List 3 occasions that you are most likely to be late.

List 3 reasons that are most likely to cause you to be late.

List 4 precautionary measures that will assist you in overcoming being late.

Structured Activity #5

What Do I Say When I Talk to You?©

Jack Kasar,
PhD, OTR/L

E. Nelson Clark,
MS, OTR/L

What Do I Say When I Talk to You?

Goal

Emphasize the importance of communicating exact information. To gain a personal awareness of how one is perceived during verbal communications.

Objectives

Participants will engage in exchange of anonymous peer evaluations of communication styles. A question/answer session may follow.

Group Size

Small classroom size group (20).

Time Frame

Thirty minutes to fill out and exchange forms, fifteen minutes discussion period.

Materials Needed

- Communication Questionnaire
- Pen/pencil

Process

1) Hand out questionnaires.
2) Instruct each individual to place their name at top.
3) Instruct individuals to hand the form to the person in front of them (or at the back of the next row) so that a "chain reaction type" process is initiated.
4) Each individual will (as accurately/fairly as possible) rate their peer on their communication styles. Continue to exchange forms until all participants have rated each form.
5) Marks are to be made in each box so that anonymity is preserved. (example: llll , lll). Please... only one mark per rater, per characteristic.
6) At the end of 30 minutes return forms to their original owners.
7) Each original owner will add up marks in each box and analyze the score for their communication style.

What Do I Say When I Talk to You?

Name:

DO I....	1 (Agree)	2	3	4 (Disagree)
Talk too fast...				
Talk too slow...				
Talk too much...				
Talk too little...				
Talk too loud...				
Talk too quiet...				
Talk too harsh... (sound angry or bossy)				
Talk too whiny.. (sound insecure or shy)				
Talk too boisterous... (brag)				
Talk too slang... (street talk)				
Talk too many additions... ("don't you know", "like..", "...okay")				

Comments/Conclusions:

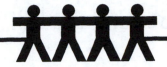

Structured
Activity #6

Seeking the Self©

Jack Kasar,
PhD, OTR/L

E. Nelson Clark,
MS, OTR/L

Seeking the Self

Goal

Being able to recognize one's own behavior and emotional responses (self-awareness) to various situations, events, and people is central and essential to health care communications. Participants should be able to begin to understand the self and develop a picture of the overall self (self-concept).

Objectives

- Recognize one's own behavior and emotional responses by completing the questionnaire and participating in group discussions.
- Receive feedback from others to see ourselves as others see us.

Group Size

The overall group should be broken down into smaller groups of six individuals per group. These subgroups should gather in small circles in order to gain as much privacy as possible.

Time Frame

- Fifteen minutes to fill out questionnaire
- Five minutes to read questionnaire by each individual and take group consensus (thirty minutes).
- Fifteen minutes for group discussion.

Materials Needed

- Questionnaire
- Pen/pencil

Process

1) Each individual completes their questionnaire. Please keep answers short but descriptive.
2) Each individual reads their questionnaire and their responses to each question. The reading individual takes a vote from the group at the end of each question. A simple show of hands whether each member of the group agrees or disagrees with the response. The reader *may not* question a member of the group as to why they agree or disagree with a statement during the voting process. Group discussions may be held about voting only if an individual agrees to respond. A vote to agree or disagree can reflect the way others perceive us by either agreeing with our own perceptions or by disagreeing with a certain perception we have of ourselves. Individuals should carefully examine the responses they give to each question and the number of agrees or disagrees to each response.

Seeking the Self

	Agree	Disagree

Appearance

When I dress up, I like to look...

My hair style is usually...

When I dress casual, I like to look...

At the beach, I feel...

My jewelry says I am...

My clothes look...

My friends tell me I look...

My ideal weight is...

Relationships

When I see someone attractive I...

In a group, I am...

With someone who has strong opinions, I usually...

If a friend tells me I am wonderful, I would...

If a friend confronts me about my problems, I...

If someone makes "fun" of me...

If I am tired and around people, I...

When I am waiting in lines (grocery store, bank, etc) I act...

If someone is staring at me, I...

When I am talking and feel ignored, I usually...

When I am ill, I usually behave...

Comments:

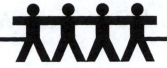

Structured Activity #7

How Much Do I Really Want It?©

Jack Kasar,
PhD, OTR/L

E. Nelson Clark,
MS, OTR/L

How Much Do I Really Want It?

Goal

Set up goals and create circumstances that will stand in the way of accomplishing these goals.

Objective

Demonstrate and assess the traits that stand in the way of goals, and examine the initiative that one must take to overcome the barriers to achievement of goals.

Group Size

A Classroom size group (10 to 30 people)

Time Frame

Twenty minutes to fill out worksheet. Thirty minutes to discuss.

Materials Needed

- Goal Setting Worksheet
- Pen/Pencil

Process

Instructions for completing "My Goal Setting Worksheet":

1) Set a goal. Be very specific. Example: "Achieve the grade of A in Anatomy". The term "good grade" in anatomy is not a specific grade and therefore not acceptable.

2) Give the goal a value in the first value column (1 thru 5). Are you capable or achieving this goal on a "routine" basis, without help? If so, give yourself the points in the second value column.

3) If you are not able to accomplish your goal on a "routine" basis, you must define exactly what you are going to do and how you are going to do it to accomplish the goal. You must also define what you will need from outside sources (person, objects, institutions) to accomplish the goal. Assign these needs a negative score. Example: Goal: Make an "A in Anatomy", Value: 5; Objects needed: Time management, tutor, sacrifice evening TV, get up early in Morning (usually sleep to 12 noon), set aside library time; etc...= -5; Strengths: family support; do not have to work for money = 2, Total Value: -3.

4) What is the total value of your goals? What is your necessary-for-achievement value? What is the difference in the two scores? Do you have enough quality changes listed to achieve your goals? What other sources do you need in order to balance the value of your goals and the value of your resources to accomplish those goals? Are your goals overvalued and your strengths undervalued or visa versa?

5) Share what you must do to change or accomplish your goals with the other participants. How can they, or someone else help you? If you can express these changes or needs, how does it feel to be able to place your goals and needs in words? If you can do this... give your score a positive value (1 thru 5).

My Goal Setting Worksheet

Name:

For the period of: Date:

Goal	Value	Sacrifices/Objects Needed	Value
1.			
2.			
3.			
4.			
5.			
6.			
7.			
Who can I share this worksheet with to help me attain these goals:	Total Value:	I am committed to taking the initiative to accomplish my GOALS: Signature:	 Total Value:

© J. Kasar and N. Clark 1998

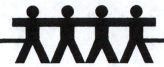

Structured
Activity #8

Who Am I and Where Am I Going?©

Jack Kasar,
PhD, OTR/L

E. Nelson Clark,
MS, OTR/L

Who Am I and Where Am I Going?

Goal

Students introduce themselves and provide their concept of helping others. They share reasons that brought them to the field of health care and provide a few goals for their professional journey.

Objectives

Participants will gain the values of empathy, cooperation, and verbal interactions by:
- Practicing data gathering
- Developing group cohesion thru gaining knowledge and understanding of others
- Listening to the opinions and experiences of others
- Practicing verbal skills

Group Size

A classroom size group (10-30).

Time Frame

Fifteen minutes to write information. Thirty minutes for sharing with others. Fifteen minutes for discussion.

Materials Needed

- 5x8 index card
- Pen/pencil

Process

1) The instructor distributes the index cards and instructs the participants to write the following information:
   - Full name and give your nickname (if appropriate)
   - A brief introduction of yourself. A few comments on likes/dislikes etc.
   - Your definition of your health care profession (PT, OT, Nursing, MA, ST, etc)
   - What got you interested in the health care field.
   - A few goals for school and your career.
   - Something another student might be able to assist you with (????)
2) The instructor directs the students to share their information with another student for about 5 minutes. This can be done by having half of the students stay stationary while the other half rotates to individuals they do not know.
3) After the students have rotated about the room for a half hour, the instructor calls time and has the students read their cards in front of the entire class. This is to illustrate that it gets easier to introduce yourself after structuring the information and then practicing it.

4) The instructor could select a student at random and ask them to give feedback, such as, who did they meet that was new to them and what was some of the information about that person that they remembered. And, were there any requests that students made (help) that they might be able to provide assistance.

Appendix

PROFESSIONAL DEVELOPMENT ASSESSMENT©

Name: _____

Evaluator (other than self): _____

Date: _____

Instructions: For each professional behavior, review the descriptors and rate 1 through 4 by circling the selected number.

Rating Scale:
1. Rarely (50% or less of the time).
2. Occasionally (50 to 75% of the time).
3. Frequently (75 to 95% of the time).
4. Consistently (95% or more of the time).

1. Dependability as demonstrated by:

a. Being on time for classes, work, meetings.	1	2	3	4
b. Handing in assignments, papers, reports and notes when due.	1	2	3	4
c. Following through with commitments and responsibilities.	1	2	3	4

Comments:

2. Professional Presentation as demonstrated by:

a. Presenting oneself in a manner that is accepted by peers, clients, and employers.	1	2	3	4
b. Using body posture and affect that communicates interest or engaged attention.	1	2	3	4
c. Displaying a positive attitude towards becoming a professional.	1	2	3	4

Comments:

3. Initiative as demonstrated by:

a. Showing an energetic, positive, and motivated manner.	1	2	3	4
b. Self-starting projects, tasks and programs.	1	2	3	4
c. Taking initiative to direct own learning.	1	2	3	4

Comments:

4. Empathy as demonstrated by:

a. Being sensitive and responding to the feelings and behaviors of others.	1	2	3	4
b. Listening to and considering the ideas and opinions of others.	1	2	3	4
c. Rendering assistance to all individuals without bias or prejudice.	1	2	3	4

Comments:

5. Cooperation as demonstrated by:

a. Working effectively with other individuals.	1	2	3	4
b. Showing consideration for the needs of the group.	1	2	3	4
c. Developing group cohesiveness by assisting in the development of the knowledge and awareness of others.	1	2	3	4

Comments:

From Kasar, J., Clark, E.N. (2000) *Developing Professional Behaviors.* Thorofare, NJ: SLACK Incorporated.
© J. Kasar, N. Clark, D. Watson, S. Pfister 1996

6. Organization as demonstrated by:

a.	Prioritizing self and tasks.	1	2	3	4
b.	Managing time and materials to meet program requirements.	1	2	3	4
c.	Using organization skills to contribute to the development of others.	1	2	3	4

Comments:

7. Clinical Reasoning as demonstrated by:

a.	Using an inquiring or questioning approach in class and clinic.	1	2	3	4
b.	Analyzing, synthesizing, and interpreting information.	1	2	3	4
c.	Giving alternative solutions to complex issues and situations.	1	2	3	4

Comments:

8. Supervisory Process as demonstrated by:

a.	Giving and receiving constructive feedback.	1	2	3	4
b.	Modifying performance in response to meaningful feedback.	1	2	3	4
c.	Operating within the scope of ones own skills and seeking guidance when needed.	1	2	3	4

Comments:

9. Verbal Communication as demonstrated by:

a.	Verbally interacting in class and clinic.	1	2	3	4
b.	Sharing perceptions and opinions with clarity and quality of content.	1	2	3	4
c.	Verbalizing opposing opinions with constructive results.	1	2	3	4

Comments:

10. Written Communication as demonstrated by:

a.	Writing clear sentences.	1	2	3	4
b.	Communicating ideas and opinions clearly and concisely in writing papers, notes, and reports.	1	2	3	4
c.	Communicating complex subject matter clearly and concisely in writing, with correct punctuation and grammar.	1	2	3	4

Comments:

From Kasar, J., Clark, E.N. (2000) *Developing Professional Behaviors.* Thorofare, NJ: SLACK Incorporated.
© J. Kasar, N. Clark, D. Watson, S. Pfister 1996

Professional Development Assessment
Rating Summary Form

Professional Behavior	Rating
1. Dependability	a._____ b._____ c._____ Total:_____
2. Professional Presentation	a._____ b._____ c._____ Total:_____
3. Initiative	a._____ b._____ c._____ Total:_____
4. Empathy	a._____ b._____ c._____ Total:_____
5. Cooperation	a._____ b._____ c._____ Total:_____
6. Organization	a._____ b._____ c._____ Total:_____
7. Clinical Reasoning	a._____ b._____ c._____ Total:_____
8. Supervisory Process	a._____ b._____ c._____ Total:_____
9. Verbal Communication	a._____ b._____ c._____ Total:_____
10. Written Communication	a._____ b._____ c._____ Total:_____

Overall Total: _____

From Kasar, J., Clark, E.N. (2000) *Developing Professional Behaviors*. Thorofare, NJ: SLACK Incorporated.
© J. Kasar, N. Clark, D. Watson, S. Pfister 1996

Professional Behaviors Feedback Form

1. Dependability

2. Professional Presentation

3. Initiative

4. Empathy

5. Cooperation

6. Organization

7. Clinical Reasoning

8. Supervisory Process

9. Verbal Communication

10. Written Communication

Index

Acceptance of medically indicated treatment, 13
Accountability, as reason for litigation, 38
Active listening, 69
Adaptability, supervisory style and, 107
Affective communication, 68
Apprentice stage, professional development, 23-24, 70, 79, 98, 140
Approach/withdraw, supervisory style and, 107
Art, and empathy, 69-70
Assessment, 145-152
    dependability, 35, 41-42
    in education, 158
    in nursing, 145
    of occupational therapists, 146
    Professional Development Assessment®, 146-151, 152, 212-214
Attitude, supervisory process and, 108-109
Autonomy, 13, 22

Be Careful What You Write©, structured activity, 180-181
Behavioral expectations
    in education, 158
    in supervision, 105-108
Behavioral style
    questionnaire, 107
    supervision and, 105
Being on Time©, structured activity, 192-193
Beneficence, ethics and, 13, 16
Body language, 46-47
Build a Better Mousetrap©, structured activity, 188-189

Change, process of, 35
Client charting, 133-134
Client information, ethics and, 14
Clinical reasoning, 7, 91-100
    components, 93
    criteria, 20
    defined, 92
    developing, 95-99
    diagnostic reasoning, 96-97
    ethics and, 16
    exercise for, 99-100
    holistic model, 93-95
    learning and teaching approaches, 161
    significance, 91-92
Clothes, professional presentation and, 46, 48-52

Codes of ethics, 13, 158
Collaboration, in a team, 76-77
Commitment, in a team, 76
Communication. See also Verbal communication; Written communication
    affective communication, 68
    basics of, 120-121
    communication style, 120
    defined, 131
    empathy, 68-70
    exercises for, 129, 141
    listening skills, 69, 127-128
    model, 119-120
    structured activities for, 180-181, 196-197, 200-201
    teamwork and, 77
    types of, 122-123
    of values, 122
Compensatory justice, 14
Competency, 13
Confidentiality, as moral principle, 14
Conflict management, supervisory process and, 110
Connotative language, 120
Continuing education, 152, 165-172
Cooperation, 7, 75-81
    criteria, 20
    developing, 79
    exercises for, 81
    foundations of, 75
    learning and teaching approaches, 161
    structured activities for, 188-189, 208-209
    in teams and groups, 75-76
Core values, 13

Decision making, ethical, 15
Democratic leadership, 111
Dentistry, dependability and, 29-32
Deontological theory, 14, 15
Dependability, 6, 29-40
    at home, 35
    case stories, 38-40
    criteria for, 20
    defined, 29-30
    developing, 32-37
    ethics and, 16
    importance of, 30-32
    learning and teaching approaches, 161

malpractice, 37-38
mentoring for, 35-36
of patients, 36
self-assessment, 35, 41-42
structured activity for, 192-193
Despair, 25
Diagnostic reasoning, 96-97
Disclosure of information, 13
Disorganization, humorousness of, 83
Distributive justice, 14
Doubt, professional development process, 22

Education
behavioral expectations in, 158
continuing education, 152, 165-172
evaluation, 152
graduate education, 172
instructional methods, 160
learning and teaching approach, 151-152, 157-162
measuring performance, 158
performance expectations, 159-160
professional education, 33, 59-60, 158
program planning, 151
Educational communication, 126
Empathy, 7, 65-71
art and, 69-70
barriers to developing, 71
case stories, 70, 71
criteria for, 20
defined, 65-66
developing, 66-70
ethics and, 16
exercises for, 73
learning and teaching approaches, 161
measuring, 66
nature of, 67
structured activity for, 200-201
Ethical codes, 13, 158
Ethical tension, 12
Ethics
codes of ethics, 13, 158
dilemmas, 11-12
law and, 14
moral development, 15
moral principles, 14
personal, 12
principles of, 13-14
problem solving, 15-16
professional, 12
professionalism and, 11-12
societal, 12
theories, 14-15
values and, 12-13
Exercises. *See also* Structured activities
attitudes and behaviors, 159
clinical reasoning, 99-100
cooperation, 81
empathy, 73
initiative, 62
organizational values, 159
professional presentation, 53
program values, 159

supervisory process, 116
verbal communication, 129
written communication, 141
Expectations of behavior, supervision, 105-108
Expert stage, professional development, 24-25, 70-71, 79, 98, 115, 140
Expressive writing, 132, 133-134
Extrinsic initiative, 57-58

Family, verbal communication within, 122-123
Feedback
educational course, 171
verbal communication, 124-125
Fidelity, 14, 16
Flexibility, supervisory process and, 108

Generativity, 24-25
Goal setting, structured activity for, 204-205
Graduate education, 172
Grooming, 47
Guilt, 22-23

Herringbone diagram, 62
Hippocratic Oath, 11
Hogan Empathy Scale, 67
Honesty, as moral principle, 14
How Much Do I Really Want It?©, structured activity, 204-205

Identity formation, 23-24
Image, 45-53. *See also* Professional presentation
Individual standards, 105
Individuation, 22
Inferiority, 23
Information-seeking interviews, 124
Informed consent, 13
Initiative, 6-7, 55-62
criteria for, 20
defined, 55
developing, 22-23, 57, 58-61
exercises for, 62
extrinsic vs. intrinsic, 57-58, 59
learning and teaching approaches, 161
significance of, 56
Institutional responsibility, 31
Integrity, 25
Intelligence, in verbal communication, 121-122
Intensity, supervisory style and, 107
Interview skills, 124
Intimacy, 24
Intonation, verbal communication, 121
Intrinsic initiative, 57-58, 59
Isolation, 24

Journal articles, writing, 139-149
Judging Books by Their Cover©, structured activity, 184-185
Justice, as ethical principle, 14

Kagan's Affective Sensitivity Scale, 67
K-W-L-S diagram, 62

Laissez-faire leadership, 111
Law, ethics and, 14
Leadership style, 110-111
Learning group, 123-124
Learning and teaching approach, 151-152, 157-162
Listening skills, 69, 127-128

Malpractice, 14, 37-38
Management style, 110-111
Medical jargon, 125
Mentorship, dependability, 35-36
Mistrust, professional development process, 21-22
Moral development, 15
Moral principles, 14
Motivation
    defined, 55
    developing, 58-60
    extrinsic vs. intrinsic, 57-58
    structured activity for, 208-209

Name tags, professional presentation, 48
Networking, 126
Nightingale Pledge, 12
Nonmaleficence, as ethical principle, 13-14
Novice stage, professional development, 21-23, 70, 79, 98, 112, 139-140
Nursing
    core values, 5, 13
    ethical dilemmas in, 11-12
    professionalism in, 5-6
    professional assessment in, 145

Occupational therapy (OT)
    core attitudes, 159
    elements of, 4
    ethical dilemmas in, 11-12
    professionalism in, 6
    self-assessment, 146
Organization, 7, 83-88
    capacity for delay, 85-86
    criteria for, 20
    defined, 83, 85
    developing, 87-88
    function of, 84-85
    lack of, 85
    learning and teaching approaches, 161
    need for, 83-84
Organizational values, exercise for, 159

Papers, writing, 135-139
Participative manager, 111
Patient compliance, 36
Patient dependability, 36
Patient/provider interaction
    communication skills, 125-126
    shared responsibility, 37
Perception, and verbal communication, 125
Persistence, supervisory style and, 107
Personal ethics, 12
Personal responsibility, of patient, 36
Physicians
    developing professionalism, 5

ethical dilemmas, 11-12
    malpractice, 14, 37-38
Pitch, verbal communication, 121
Prejudice, in verbal communication, 121-122
Privacy, as moral principle, 14
Problem solving, ethical, 15-16
Problem-solving group, 123-124
Problem-solving interviews, 124
Procedural justice, 14
Procrastination, 84
Profession, defined, 4
Professional behaviors, 3, 6-7, 19
    assessment, 145-152
    clinical reasoning, 7, 20, 91-100
    cooperation, 7, 20, 75-81
    criteria for, 20
    dependability, 6, 20, 29-40
    developing, 151-152, 161
    empathy, 7, 16, 20, 65-71
    ethics and, 16
    exercises. See Exercises
    initiative, 6-7, 20, 22-23, 55-62
    learning and teaching approaches, 161
    organization, 7, 20, 83-88
    professional presentation, 6, 20, 45-53
    structured activities. See Structured activities
    supervisory process, 7, 16, 20, 103-116
    verbal communication, 7, 20, 119-128
    written communication, 7, 20, 131-141
Professional codes of ethics, 13
Professional development, stages of, 19-25, 79, 98, 112, 115, 139-140
Professional Development Assessment®, 146-151, 152, 212-214
Professional education, 33, 59-60, 158. See also Education
Professional ethics, 12
Professionalism, 3-7
    criteria for, 19
    defined, 32-33
    developing, 5, 16
    ethics and, 11-12, 16
    name tags and, 48
    in nursing, 5-6
    in occupational therapy, 6
Professionalism Inventory, 145
Professional Nursing Behavior Instrument, 145
Professional practice, defined, 4
Professional presentation, 6, 45-53
    blink test for, 52
    body language, 46-47
    clothing, 46, 48-52
    criteria for, 20
    ethics and, 16
    exercises for, 53
    grooming, 47
    learning and teaching approaches, 161
    name tags and, 48
    structured activity for, 184-185
Professional Self Description Form, 146
Program values, exercise for, 159
Publishing, writing for, 139-149

Reasoning, clinical. *See* Clinical reasoning
Refusal of medically indicated treatment, 13
Relationships, moral principles related to, 14
Respect, supervisory process and, 109
Responsibility, 29, 31
Role confusion, 23-24
Role models, 35-36, 152
Rules of consent, 14

Sanctions, 14
Seeking the Self©, structured activity, 200-201
Self-actualization, 57
Self-assessment. *See* Assessment
Self-doubt, professional development process, 22
Self-esteem, professional development process, 22
Service learning, 69
Shame, professional development process, 22
Sincerity, in verbal communication, 122
SOAP note, 133, 134
Social interaction, verbal communication, 124
Societal ethics, 12
SOLER (acronym), 69
Stagnation, 24-25
Standards of care, as reason for litigation, 38
Structured activities. *See also* Exercises
    Be Careful What You Write©, 180-181
    Being on Time©, 192-193
    Build a Better Mousetrap©, 188-189
    How Much Do I Really Want It?©, 204-205
    Judging Books by Their Cover©, 184-185
    Seeking the Self©, 200-201
    What Do I Say When I Talk to You?©, 196-197
    Who Am I and Where Am I Going?©, 208-209
Supervision. *See also* Supervisory process
    amount of, 110
    behavioral traits and, 105, 106
    defined, 103
    exercise for, 116
    expectations of behavior, 105-108
    learning, 104-108
    management style, 110-111
    needs and, 104-105
    skill levels, 111-115
Supervisory process, 7, 16, 103-116. *See also* Supervision
    criteria for, 20
    defined, 103
    exercises for, 116
    learning and teaching approaches, 161
Supervisory qualities, 108-110
Support, supervisory process and, 109
Sympathy, 65

Teams
    career development and, 79
    communication group process, 123-124
    components of success, 75-76
    developing skills, 75-76, 79
    roles of members, 78
    structured activity for, 188-189
    verbal communication within, 123
Teleological theory, 14, 15
Time management, 33-34

Training. *See* Education
Transactional writing, 132, 135-139
Trust
    dependability as, 31-32
    professional development process, 21-22
    supervisory process and, 109
Truth, as moral principle, 14

Utilitarianism, 15

Values
    communication of, 122
    ethics and, 12-13
Venn diagram, 61
Veracity, as moral principle, 14
Verbal communication, 7, 119-129
    criteria for, 20
    defined, 119
    developing awareness, 127-129
    educational communication, 126
    ethics and, 16
    exercise for, 129
    feedback, 124-125
    in groups, 123-124
    in health care, 125-126
    "I" messages, 125
    inherent qualities, 120
    intelligence and, 121-122
    interviews, 124
    learning and teaching approaches, 161
    listening skills, 127-128
    medical jargon, 125
    model, 119-120
    openness, 125
    with patients, 125-126
    perception and, 125
    personal style and, 120
    pitch and intonation, 121
    prejudice and, 121-122
    with professionals, 126
    social interaction, 124
    structured activities for, 196-197, 208-209
    of values, 122
    within family, 122-123

What Do I Say When I Talk to You?©, structured activity, 196-197
Who Am I and Where Am I Going?©, structured activity, 208-209
Written communication, 7, 131-141
    client charting, 133-134
    criteria for, 20
    defined, 131
    developing, 132-133
    ethics and, 16
    exercise for, 141
    expressive writing, 132-134
    learning and teaching approaches, 161
    significance, 131-132
    structured activity for, 180-181
    transactional writing, 132, 135-139